COLOR ATLAS OF
ORAL
MANIFESTATIONS OF
AIDS

Publisher

B.C. Decker Inc
3228 South Service Road
Burlington, Ontario   L7N 3H8

B.C. Decker Inc
320 Walnut Street
Suite 400
Philadelphia, Pennsylvania   19106

Sales and Distribution

United States and Puerto Rico
The C.V. Mosby Company
11830 Westline Industrial Drive
Saint Louis, Missouri   63146

Canada
McAinsh & Co. Ltd.
2760 Old Leslie Street
Willowdale, Ontario   M2K 2X5

Australia
McGraw-Hill Book Company Australia Pty. Ltd.
4 Barcoo Street
Roseville East 2069
New South Wales, Australia

Brazil
Editora McGraw-Hill do Brasil, Ltda.
rua Tabapua, 1.105, Itaim-Bibi
Sao Paulo, S.P. Brasil

Colombia
Interamericana/McGraw-Hill de Colombia, S.A.
Apartado Aereo 81078
Bogota, D.E. Colombia

Europe
McGraw-Hill Book Company GmbH
Lademannbogen 136
D-2000 Hamburg 63
West Germany

France
MEDSI/McGraw-Hill
6, avenue Daniel Lesueur
75007 Paris, France

Hong Kong and China
McGraw-Hill Book Company
Suite 618, Ocean Centre
5 Canton Road
Tsimshatsui, Kowloon
Hong Kong

India
Tata McGraw-Hill Publishing Company, Ltd.
12/4 Asaf Ali Road, 3rd Floor
New Delhi 110002, India

Indonesia
P.O. Box 122/JAT
Jakarta, 1300 Indonesia

Italy
McGraw-Hill Libri Italia, s.r.l.
Piazza Emilia, 5
I-20129 Milano MI
Italy

Japan
Igaku-Shoin Ltd.
Tokyo International P.O. Box 5063
1-28-36 Hongo, Bunkyo-ku,
Tokyo 113, Japan

Korea
C.P.O. Box 10583
Seoul, Korea

Malaysia
No. 8 Jalan SS 7/6B
Kelana Jaya
47301 Petaling Jaya
Selangor, Malaysia

Mexico
Interamericana/McGraw-Hill de Mexico, S.A. de C.V.
Cedro 512, Colonia Atlampa
(Apartado Postal 26370)
06450 Mexico, D.F., Mexico

New Zealand
McGraw-Hill Book Co. New Zealand Ltd.
5 Joval Place, Wiri
Manukau City, New Zealand

Panama
Editorial McGraw-Hill Latinoamericana, S.A.
Apartado Postal 2036
Zona Libre de Colon
Colon, Republica de Panama

Portugal
Editora McGraw-Hill de Portugal, Ltda.
Rua Rosa Damasceno 11A–B
1900 Lisboa, Portugal

South Africa
Libriger Book Distributors
Warehouse Number 8
"Die Ou Looiery"
Tannery Road
Hamilton, Bloemfontein 9300

Southeast Asia
McGraw-Hill Book Co.
348 Jalan Boon Lay
Jurong, Singapore 2261

Spain
McGraw-Hill/Interamericana de Espana, S.A.
Manuel Ferrero, 13
28020 Madrid, Spain

Taiwan
P.O. Box 87–601
Taipei, Taiwan

Thailand
632/5 Phaholyothin Road
Sapan Kwai
Bangkok 10400
Thailand

United Kingdom, Middle East and Africa
McGraw-Hill Book Company (U.K.) Ltd.
Shoppenhangers Road
Maidenhead, Berkshire
SL6 2QL England

Venezuela
McGraw-Hill/Interamericana, C.A.
2da. calle Bello Monte
(entre avenida Casanova y Sabana Grande)
Apartado Aereo 50785
Caracas 1050, Venezuela

NOTICE

The authors and publisher have made every effort to ensure that the patient care recommended herein, including choice of drugs and drug dosages, is in accord with the accepted standards and practice at the time of publication. However, since research and regulation constantly change clinical standards, the reader is urged to check the product information sheet included in the package of each drug, which includes recommended doses, warnings, and contraindications. This is particularly important with new or infrequently used drugs.

Color Atlas of Oral Manifestations of AIDS

ISBN 1-55664-199-0

Library of Congress catalog card number: 89–50851

10 9 8 7 6 5 4 3 2 1

COLOR ATLAS OF
ORAL
MANIFESTATIONS OF
AIDS

SOL SILVERMAN JR., M.A., D.D.S.

Professor and Chairman of Oral Medicine
School of Dentistry
University of California
San Francisco, California

1989
B.C. Decker • Toronto • Philadelphia

Preface

Knowingly and unknowingly, clinicians are treating patients who are infected with the AIDS virus. This *Color Atlas of Oral Manifestations of AIDS* is designed to give clinicians a quick, updated, and practical approach to diagnosing and managing oral lesions associated with human immunodeficiency virus (HIV) infection. Additionally, the atlas is intended to assist the clinician in suspecting HIV infection when a patient's status is unknown.

Utilizing brief and concise text, this atlas also gives an overview of the epidemiology of the AIDS pandemic, provides insight into the biology of HIV infection, and describes progression of HIV infection involving opportunistic infections, malignancies, autoimmune conditions, and a variety of as yet unclassified manifestations. References are current, are organized by topic for effective review, and reflect recent developments and views, supportive studies, and author experience.

The main and unique emphasis lies in a selection of photographs that depicts the following: diverse appearances of the many oral lesions to help in the differential diagnosis; the many treatment modalities and results; the successful outcomes that can be planned and achieved; and progression of disease so that eventual clinical complications and management problems, oral health counseling, and appropriate referrals can be realistically anticipated.

Sol Silverman Jr.
June, 1989

Contents

1

THE NATURE OF HIV INFECTION

EPIDEMIOLOGY AND BIOLOGY

The Acquired Immunodeficiency Syndrome (AIDS) epidemic, unequivocally caused by the human immunodeficiency virus (HIV), continues on without any end in sight. At this time there are many reasons to support this bleak outlook.

1. AIDS is a worldwide pandemic, with essentially all countries in the world reporting HIV-infected persons and cases of AIDS.

2. It is estimated that the AIDS virus (HIV) probably already has infected in excess of 10 million men and women throughout the world. At any stage following HIV infection, HIV-infected individuals may be capable of transmitting the virus to sex partners (semen, vaginal fluid), by blood transfer (contaminated needles, transfusions), or through birth (from an infected mother). In the United States up to 1.5 million Americans are estimated to be HIV-infected.

3. HIV-infected persons are often asymptomatic for a prolonged period of time and unaware of being either infected or a carrier.

4. Most, if not all, HIV positive individuals are infected for life; and while it still remains inconclusive, most may eventually develop AIDS. Incubation periods can exist for many years, with extrapolation models indicating a median time of more than 8 years. HIV infection initiates a diverse continuum of disease: It begins in some with a self-limiting retroviral sickness, while in all there is an asymptomatic phase; this is followed by a period of quite variable signs and/or symptoms (AIDS related complex, ARC); and finally HIV infection ends in the terminal phase of AIDS, that is the development of specific opportunistic infections and malignancies which fall within the Centers for Disease Control definitions of AIDS.

5. Viral gene mutations, which induce variations in protein composition, occur frequently in this retrovirus. The rate of mutation appears to be greater than in any other virus that infects mankind. Thus, considerable heterogenicity exists among isolates. This at least in part accounts for the diversity of signs and symptoms and the emergence of "new" strains. Additionally, another similar lethal retrovirus, HIV-2, has been well described in Africa, Europe, and the United States. Furthermore, mutations create uncertainties regarding HIV virulence, hence adding uncertainties as to the success of eventual vaccines and treatment modalities.

TRANSMISSION AND PROGRESSION

At present all of the influences regarding risks of transmission and infectivity are not completely clear. When a host is exposed to HIV, infection depends upon many known and some speculated factors which include the following: Concentration of virus; multiple exposures; stimulation and effectiveness of host neutralizing antibodies; abundance of cell-surface receptors, such as CD4 protein; and host co-factors, such as other microbial infections that may aid HIV replication. While the use of hallucinogens appears to be a risk factor also, this may be on the basis of a behavioral influence (sexual promiscuity and insensitivity to the use of barrier techniques).

Eventually, or at least in most HIV-infected individuals, a copy of the viral genome, which has been incorporated as an integral and permanent component of the infected hosts nuclear DNA (by viral reverse transcriptase), will start copying itself. This viral replication activity leads to an exacerbation of the infection, with progressive immunosuppression and a subsequent cascade of HIV manifestations. The co-factors necessary for the activation and intensity of viral replication remain an enigma.

As the virus reproduces itself, more host cells are infected, particularly helper-inducer lymphocytes (T4), which appear to contain most of the cell surface receptors that allow further cell invasion and flare the severity of the infection. This is of particular significance, since the T4 helper-inducer lymphocyte is the key modulator of the immune system, primarily through its chemical controls (lymphokines/cytokines) of B lymphocyte and macrophage activities. As the T4 lymphocytes are reduced in number through progressive infection and cell destruction, the host is rendered more susceptible to opportunistic infections and malignancies. It should also be pointed out that, during asymptomatic phases, HIV-infected lymphocytes and free virus can be found, and hence hosts are still potentially infectious in these periods.

DEMOGRAPHICS

The distribution of individuals infected with HIV throughout the world varies according to initial time of geographic exposure to the virus, habits, customs, socioeconomic conditions, and reporting systems. In some African countries the rate of HIV infection seems to be the highest. The largest number of AIDS cases has been reported in the United States. It is most commonly found in homosexual and bisexual men, but this pattern is slowly changing. In underdeveloped countries AIDS is common in women, probably because of prostitution, low use of barrier techniques, genital diseases, and anal intercourse. AIDS is firmly established in the heterosexual population, mainly in intravenous drug abusers.

In the United States approximately 68 percent of reported AIDS cases occur in homosexual or bisexual men, 22 percent in heterosexual men (which includes blood transfusion victims), about 8 percent in women (most of whom are intravenous drug abusers and/or prostitutes), and about 2 percent in children and adolescents. It is estimated that about 30 percent of HIV positive pregnant women give birth to infected offspring. HIV infection is rare in non-high risk groups, occurring primarily in either men or women who are not aware of an infected sex partner, by recipients of blood transfusions that contain the virus, and by accidental exposure to contaminated blood by needle penetration or injury (Chapter 2).

There are definite ethnic influences that again appear to be related to socioeconomic and educational bases. In the United States about 60 percent of the adult victims are white males, primarily between the ages of 20 to 40 years; however, in women and intravenous drug abusers who have developed AIDS, blacks and Hispanics make up approximately 70 percent of that group; and in those AIDS patients under the age of 13, 75 percent are black and Hispanic. In other countries, gender, distribution, and manifestations vary. Again, the diversities are based on habits, customs, education, socioeconomic factors, and availability of treatment.

SURVIVAL

AIDS is essentially a 100 percent lethal disease, and it is thought, but not proven, that most HIV-infected individuals will eventually develop AIDS and not survive this lethal disease. The cause of death is usually from an opportunistic infection or malignancy. The most frequent infection and cause of death in AIDS is related to *Pneumocystis carinii* pneumonia and respiratory failure. There is very little evidence to support the concept that HIV infection is reversible.

Survival varies considerably, being dependent upon disease(s) at diagnosis, age, race, risk group, longevity of HIV infection, availability of treatment, and unidentified-variable biologic host factors. However, most HIV-infected patients die within two years after the definitive diagnosis of AIDS is established. There are some victims that live for many years with varying qualities of life. Certain biologic factors, such as lowered number of T4 lymphocytes, increase in P24 (core protein) antigenemia, and increased beta-2 microglobulin levels, appear to be independent predictors of progression to AIDS and therefore, to limited survival. Undoubtedly, behavioral factors play an important role. These would include compliance with therapeutic regimes, protected sexual activity, and altering detrimental habits, such as drug usage.

REFERENCES

Epidemiology and Biology

Brookmeyer R, Gail MH, Polk BF. The prevalent cohort study and the acquired immunodeficiency syndrome. Am J Epidemiol 1987; 126:14-24.

Centers for Disease Control. Revision of the CDC surveillance case definition for acquired immunodeficiency syndrome. MMWR 1987; 36 (suppl no. IS): 3-15.

Centers for Disease Control. Human immunodeficiency virus infection in the United States: a review of current knowledge. MMWR 1987; 36 (suppl. no. S-6): 1-48.

Clavel F, Mansinho K, Charmaret S, et al. Human immunodeficiency virus type 2 infection associated with AIDS in West Africa. N Engl J Med 1987; 316:1180-1185.

Evans AS. Does HIV cause AIDS? An historical perspective. JAIDS 1989; 2:107-113.

Gallo RC. HIV–the cause of AIDS: An overview on its biology, mechanisms of disease induction, and our attempts to control it. JAIDS 1988; 1:521-535.

Karon JM, Dondero TJ, Curran JW. The projected incidence of AIDS and estimated prevalence of HIV infection in the United States. JAIDS 1988; 1:542-550.

Quinn TC, Zacarias FRK, St. John RK. AIDS in The Americas. An emerging public health crisis. N Engl J Med 1989; 320:1005-1007.

Transmission and Progression

Centers for Disease Control. Update: serologic testing for antibody to human immunodeficiency virus. MMWR 1988; 37:833-845.

Centers for Disease Control. Condoms for prevention of sexually transmitted diseases. MMWR 1988; 37:133-137.

Dinarello CA, Mier JW. Current concepts. Lymphokines. N Engl J Med 1988; 317:940-945.

Francis DP, Chin J. The prevention of acquired immunodeficiency syndrome in the United States. JAMA 1987; 257:1357-1366.

Haseltine WA. Replication and pathogenesis of the AIDS virus. JAIDS 1988; 1:241-245.

Ho DD, Pomerantz RJ, Kaplan JC. Pathogenesis of infection with human immunodeficiency virus. N Engl J Med 1987; 317:278-286.

Holmes KK, Kreiss J. Heterosexual transmission of human immunodeficiency virus: overview of a neglected aspect of the AIDS epidemic. JAIDS 1988; 1:602-610.

Institute of Medicine/National Academy of Sciences. Confronting AIDS: Update 1988. Executive summary. JAIDS 1988; 1:173-186.

Lui K-J, Darrow WW, Rutherford GW. A model-based estimate of the mean incubation period for AIDS in homosexual men. Science 1988; 240:1333-1335.

Medley GF, Anerson RM, Cox DR, Billard L. Incubation period of AIDS in patients infected via blood transfusion. Nature 1987; 328:719-721.

Quinn TC, Piot P, McCormick JB, et al. Serologic and immunologic studies in patients with AIDS in North America and Africa. The potential role of infectious agents as cofactors in human immunodeficiency virus infection. JAMA 1987; 257:2617-2621.

Sande MA. Transmission of AIDS. The case against casual contagion. N Engl J Med 1986; 314:380-382.

Taylor JMG, Fahey JL, Detals R, Giorgi JV. CD4 percentage, CD4 number, and CD4: CD88 ratio in HIV infection: Which to use and how to use. JAIDS 1989; 2:114-124.

Demographics

Centers for Disease Control. Antibody to human immunodeficiency virus in female prostitutes. MMWR 1987; 36:157–161.

Centers for Disease Control. Quarterly report to the domestic policy council on the prevalence and rate of spread of HIV and AIDS. MMWR 1988; 37:551–559.

Centers for Disease Control. Number of sex partners and potential risk of sexual exposure to human immunodeficiency virus. MMWR 1988; 37:567–568.

Centers for Disease Control. Trends in human immunodeficiency virus infection among civilian applicants for military service—United States, October 1986-March 1988. MMWR 1988; 37:677–679.

Curran JW, Jaffe HW, Hardy AM, et al. Epidemiology of HIV infection and AIDS in the United States. Science 1988; 239:610–615.

Padian HS. Heterosexual transmission of acquired immunodeficiency syndromes: international perspectives and national projections. Rev Infect Dis 1987; 9:947–960.

Selik RM, Castro KG, Pappaioanou M. Distribution of AIDS cases, by racial/ethnic group and exposure category, United States, June 1, 1981—July 4, 1988. MMWR 1988; 37 (suppl no. ss-3):1–10.

Survival

Anderson RM. The role of mathematical models in the study of HIV transmission and the epidemiology of AIDS. JAIDS 1988; 1:241–256.

MacDonell KB, Chmiel JS, Goldsmith J, et al. Prognostic usefulness of the Walter Reed staging classification for HIV infection. JAIDS 1988; 1:367–374.

Moss AR, Bacchetti I, Osmond D, et al. Seropositivity for HIV and the development of AIDS or AIDS related condition: three year follow up of the San Francisco General Hospital cohort. Br Med J 1988; 296:745–750.

Polk B, Fox R, Brookmeyer R, et al. Predictors of the acquired immunodeficiency syndrome developing in a cohort of seropositive homosexual men. N Engl J Med 1987; 316:61–66.

Rothenberg R, Woelfel M, Stoneburner R, et al. Survival with the acquired immunodeficiency syndrome. Experience with 5933 cases in New York City. N Engl J Med 1987; 317:1297–1302.

2

ORAL MANIFESTATIONS OF HIV INFECTION

ROLE OF PROFESSIONALS

Knowledge in HIV infection has become a critically important requirement for professionals who are responsible for oral health care delivery. This role and need for combined education and understanding is based upon the following:

1. HIV infected individuals actively seek consultation and care for oral health. Often patients themselves do not know their infectivity status; and knowingly or unknowingly regarding HIV status, treatment is being given.

2. Many times oral complaints and findings are the first signs and/or symptoms of HIV infection, or even AIDS. History taking, examination, differential diagnosis, and patient referral have taken on new dimensions.

3. Often the oral lesions associated with HIV infection interfere sufficiently with well-being to require treatment, which frequently is best provided by those trained in oral health care services.

4. Persistence or re-emergence of oral diseases may reflect therapeutic resistance and progression of generalized disease.

5. Possibilities of transmission to those having patient contact, office workers, and patients have created great emotional concerns, as well as the impact on office infectious disease control techniques and costs.

6. Ethical and legal guidelines mandate against discriminations and biases regarding availability and performance of services.

7. It should also be remembered that in addition to HIV, many other microorganisms may pose a threat, such as hepatitis B virus and herpes-family viruses.

INFECTIVITY, RISKS, GUIDELINES

Hepatitis B virus (HBV) has been used as a standard for risks and guidelines because that epidemic has been recognized for many decades. HBV poses a risk of transmission for health care workers, and also has significance since HBV carriers represent the same risk groups for HIV infectivity.

However, compared to HBV, HIV has a relatively low virulence. But, quite opposite from HBV, HIV is essentially 100 percent lethal and there is neither an effective vaccine nor a curative treatment. Thus, in addition to the biologic gravity of the disease, there is a great emotional fear of the HIV epidemic which transcends all phases of our society, that is, social, economic, scientific, political, and legal. Based on both the biological aspects and emotional concerns surrounding HIV infection and AIDS, mandatory guidelines have been developed to insure adequate protection for health care workers and the public. These guidelines include a variety of barrier techniques, proper disinfection and sterilization, and controls for cross-contamination.

Barrier techniques include the use of gloves for all patient contact (new gloves for each patient), eye protection, masks when spray and aerosolization are expected, and gowns. While heat sterilization is optimal and recommended when possible, proper use of disinfectant solutions can give adequate protection. Following manufacturers' guidelines for dilution, temperature, freshness, and time can accomplish disinfection as well as sterilization under appropriate conditions. Cross-contamination prevention entails care of equipment and furniture, use of disposable items when possible, care while taking radiographs, garbage disposal regulations, and proper handling of impressions and models. Understanding and use of the disinfectant solutions are critical in this sphere of operation. Obviously techniques for needle disposal, protection during instrument handling and cleaning, and managing spills are important.

While history taking is important, often "protected" and incorrect responses will occur. When the information is complete and accurate, certain past diseases may indicate a risk group member. Most commonly a history of venereal disease or hepatitis reflects behavior that increases the risk for HIV exposure. Addictive/habituating drug usage and heavy alcohol consumption should also arouse suspicion.

Other rather common findings that may be indicative of risks for HIV infection include unexplained weight loss, diarrhea, fevers, and night sweats. Complaints of memory loss or forgetfulness are of significance. It must be remembered that HIV is also neurotropic; about 40 percent of all HIV-infected individuals will develop central nervous system involvement during the course of their disease, and in 10 percent this affliction may be the first sign of infection. Frequent colds and sore throats, malaise, and fatigability may be suspicious indicators.

The scarce findings of HIV seroconversion and AIDS amongst non-high risk health care workers (primarily no history of homosexuality, bisexuality, intravenous drug abuse, or known HIV-positive sex partner) indicate that there is an extremely low risk for transmission through professional services or accidental injuries. There is no compelling evidence that HIV is transmitted by routes other than sexual activity, blood transfer, or birth from HIV-positive mother. Therefore, the probability of infection among health care workers from work-associated functions approaches zero, even taking accidents and injuries (primarily needle sticks and splashes) into consideration. However, since there is a very, very small possibility despite the low probability, to follow protective infectious disease control guidelines is prudent, essential, and mandatory.

In summary, fears of offering treatment to those infected should be abated based on the relatively low virulence and known transmission routes of HIV, and the very rare occurrence in non-high risk health care workers. In addition, saliva has been shown to be an inefficient carrier of the AIDS virus, both in frequency and concentrations. Furthermore, there appears to be a protein inhibitory factor(s) in saliva that may account for this phenomena, possibly even in the presence of saliva contaminated with infected blood. If these findings were not true, many more health professionals in non-high risk groups, who for years have not taken proper precautions, would be carriers or victims of the AIDS virus.

DIFFERENTIAL DIAGNOSIS OF ORAL MANIFESTATIONS

It has been shown repeatedly that oral lesions have great significance as possibly the first sign and/or symptom of HIV infection, the progression of HIV disease, and being a cause of dysfunction, pain, and unacceptable appearance. Therefore, recognition, diagnosis, and management of AIDS-associated oral diseases are important components in education, treatment and research in the AIDS epidemic.

As immune competence decreases, a spectrum of oral and paraoral pathology may appear, and frequently does. These include viral, bacterial and fungal opportunistic infections, malignancies, auto-immune lesions, and other non-classifiable abnormalities. The diversifications in appearance, frequency, and time of occurrence are not clearly understood, but are obviously due to complex and variable co-factors. As stated already, most of these lesions have implications regarding diagnosis of HIV infection, prognosis, and quality of life.

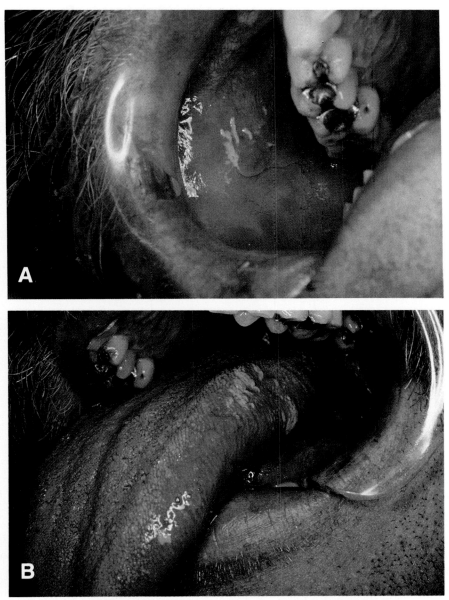

Figure 2.1   This 28 year old bisexual man reported to the clinic for routine dental care. He acknowledged a history of gonorrhea and hepatitis B. Clinical examination revealed: (1) asymptomatic surface white lesions on the buccal mucosa (A) which were confirmed as candidal colonies; and (2) white lesions on the lateral border of the tongue (B) which were confirmed as "hairy leukoplakia" (Chapters 3 and 4). After appropriate counseling, serologic testing indicated that the patient was HIV infected.

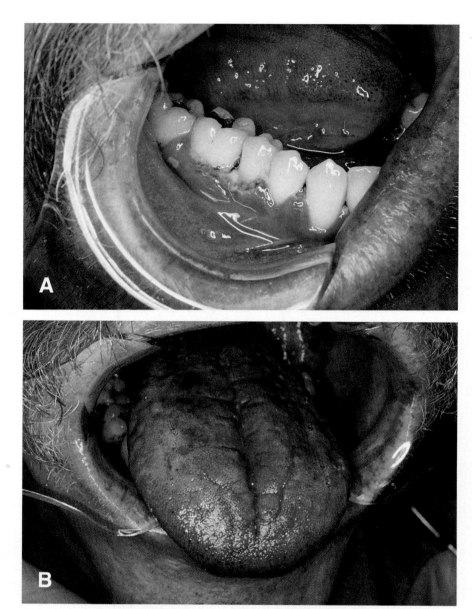

Figure 2.2   This 30 year old homosexual male patient reported to our clinic because of a painful and unexplainable acute necrotizing ulcerative gingivitis (A). He had a history of presently controlled venereal disease and hepatitis (forms unknown). He occasionally smoked marijuana. Oral examination also revealed glossitis that was only mildly irritable (B). This was confirmed as due to candidiasis. Three months later he developed a cough, and *Pneumocystis carinii* pneumonia was diagnosed. He died of AIDS 1 year later.

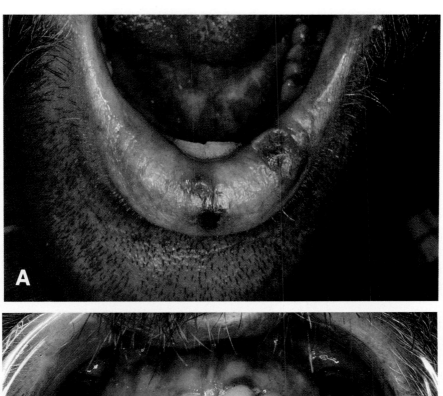

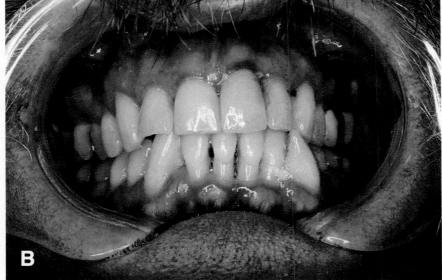

Figure 2.3   This 31 year old homosexual patient sought consultation because of an increase in frequency and severity of recurrent cold sores associated with his lower lip (A). Examination also revealed a premature periodontosis (B). With the patient's consent and appropriate orientation, a serologic test proved to be HIV positive. Since an asymptomatic Kaposi's sarcoma of the gingiva (labial marginal gingiva, upper left central incisor) was also coincidentally diagnosed, the patient could already be classified as having AIDS.

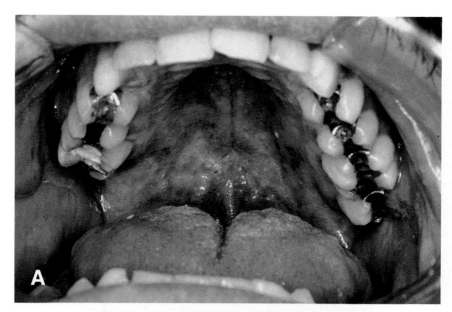

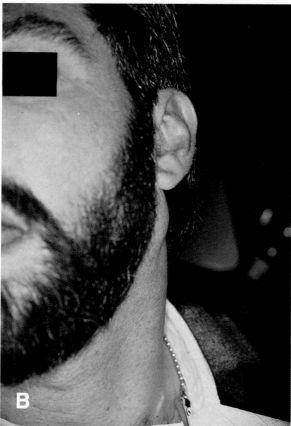

Figure 2.4 A 31 year old bisexual male sought consultation because of palatal "irritation." His medical history was negative except for a past bout with venereal disease, recent fatigability, and slight weight loss. Clinical examination revealed the erythematous form of candidiasis on his palate (A), and a "lump" in the neck (B), which was shown to be idiopathic benign lymphadenopathy (manifestation of the "gay lymph node syndrome"). This prompted suspicion of immunosuppression, confirmed by positive HIV seroantibodies.

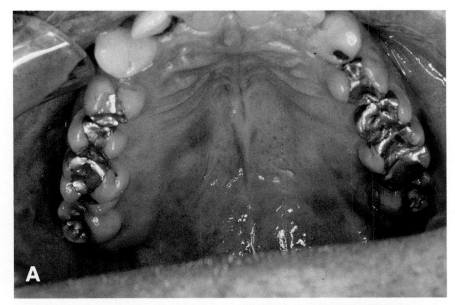

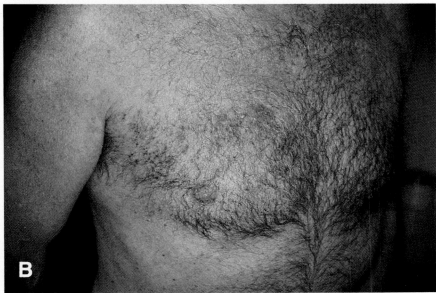

Figure 2.5   This 40 year old homosexual male sought consultation because of a palatal discomfort. He had no other complaints except for "forgetfulness" and "hand tremors." Medical history was positive for venereal disease and occasional diarrhea due to parasitic infections. Clinical examination revealed palatal discolorations that would not blanch upon pressure (A). A palatal biopsy proved the lesions to be Kaposi's sarcoma, and serology demonstrated HIV antibodies. During the next 6 months before his death, he developed zoster (B), erythema multiforme, progressive weakness, weight loss, and obvious leukoencephalopathy (due to central nervous system HIV infection).

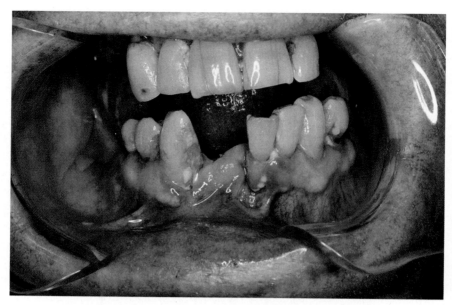

Figure 2.6   This 68 year old man was referred because of progressive periodontal disease, oral pain, anorexia, dysgeusia, and loss of weight of 4 months duration. Except for past angina and hypertension, the patient's medical history was negative. Because of coronary artery occlusions, bypass surgery with multiple transfusions was performed 4 years previously. He also had a mild mucosal candidiasis and HIV testing was positive. Since there was no other high risk activity revealed, it was presumed that HIV infection was derived from the blood transfusion.

REFERENCES

Role of Professionals

Gerbert B, Maguire B, Badner V, et al. Changing dentists' knowledge, attitudes, and behaviors relating to AIDS: a controlled educational intervention. J Am Dent Assoc 1988; 116:851–854.

Health and Public Policy Committee, American College of Physicians and the Infectious Diseases Society of America. The acquired immunodeficiency syndrome (AIDS) and infection with the human immunodeficiency virus (HIV). Ann Intern Med 1988; 108:460–469.

Logan MK. Legal implications of infectious disease in the dental office. J Am Dent Assoc 1987; 115:850–854.

Pindborg JJ. Classification of oral lesions associated with HIV infection. Oral Surg Oral Med Oral Pathol 1989; 67:292–295.

Silverman S Jr, Migliorati CA, Lozada-Nur F. Oral findings in people with or at high risk for AIDS: a study of 375 homosexual males. J Am Dent Assoc 1986; 112:187–192.

Infectivity, Risks, Guidelines

ADA Reports. Infection control recommendations for the dental office and the dental laboratory. J Am Dent Assoc 1988; 116:241–248.

ADA Research Institute, Department of Toxicology. Infectious hazards for both dental personnel and patients in the operatory. J Am Dent Assoc 1988; 117:374.

Archibald DW, Barr CE, Torosian JP, McLane MF. Secretory IgA antibodies to human immunodeficiency virus in the parotid saliva of patients with AIDS and AIDS-related complex. J Infect Dis 1987; 165:793–796.

Bolski E, Hunt RJ. The prevalence of AIDS-associated oral lesions in a cohort of patients with hemophilia. Oral Surg Oral Med Oral Pathol 1988; 65:406–410.

Castro KG, Lifson AR, White CR, et al. Investigations of AIDS patients with no previously identified risk factors. JAMA 1988, 259:1338–1342.

Centers for Disease Control. Recommendations for prevention of HIV transmission in health care settings. MMWR 1987, 36 (suppl no. 2S):3–18.

Centers for Disease Control. Agent summary statement for human immunodeficiency viruses (HIVs) including HTLV-III, LAV, HIV-1, and HIV-2. MMWR 1988; 37:1–18.

Centers for Disease Control. Update: acquired immunodeficiency syndrome and human immunodeficiency virus infection among health-care workers. MMWR 1988; 37:229–239.

Dobloug JH, Gerner NW, Hurlen B, et al. HIV and hepatitis B infection in an international cohort of dental hygienists. Scand J Dent Res 1988; 96:448–450.

Flynn NM, Pollet SM, VanHorne JR, et al. Absence of HIV antibody among dental professionals exposed to infected patients. West J Med 1987; 146:439–442.

Fox PC, Wolff A, Yeh C-K, et al. Saliva inhibits HIV-1 infectivity. JADA 1988; 116:635–637.

Gerberding JL, Greene J. AIDS update. Occupational exposure. Human immunodeficiency virus: risks to health care workers and review of infection control guidelines. Calif Dent Assoc J 1987; 15:48–51.

Gerberding JL, Bryant-LeBlanc CE, Nelson K, et al. Risk of transmitting the human immunodeficiency virus, cytomegalovirus, and hepatitis B virus to health care workers exposed to patients with AIDS and AIDS-related conditions. J Infect Dis 1987; 156:1–8.

Verrusio CA. Risk of transmission of the human immunodeficiency virus to health care workers exposed to HIV-infected patients: a review. JADA 1989; 118:339–342.

3

FUNGAL INFECTIONS: Candidiasis

SIGNIFICANCE

Candidal fungi are commonly found as part of the oral microbial flora in HIV infected persons. Therefore, it is not surprising that candidal overgrowth is the most common infection in HIV positive individuals. Recognition is important since oral candidiasis may have a significant bearing on a patient's oral and general health. Oral candidiasis may or may not be recognized by the host; however, identification and management have a significant impact on the patient's well-being for the following reasons:

1. Oral candidiasis may be the first sign and/or symptom of HIV infection.

2. If a known HIV positive patient has oral candidiasis, the prognosis for extended survival appears to be diminished.

3. Oral candidiasis usually produces bothersome symptoms of discomfort or pain, halitosis, and dysgeusia, all of which require some form of treatment.

4. Oral candidiasis may aggravate an already compromised immune system by further suppressing T-lymphocyte functions.

5. Oral candidiasis may serve as a focus for candidal colonization at other sites such as the esophagus or respiratory tract; however, systemic candidiasis in HIV infected individuals is extremely rare.

DIAGNOSIS

It is obvious then that recognition and treatment of oral candidiasis is important. Diagnosis can be difficult, since oral candidiasis has quite variable manifestations, which include: various shapes, sizes, and forms of white mucosal-surface fungal colonies; diverse patterns of mucosal erythema; combinations of red and white changes; and even erosive lesions. Angular cheilitis often accompanies the intra-oral infection (Figures 3.1–3.7).

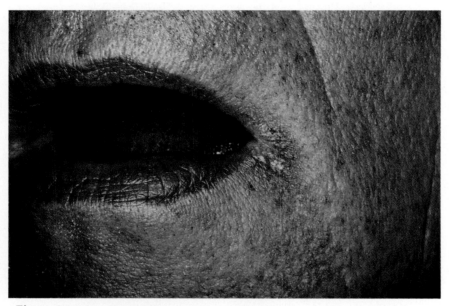

Figure 3.1 Angular cheilitis in a 60 year old homosexual male. This was the first sign of oral candidiasis and HIV infection, the latter proved by positive serology.

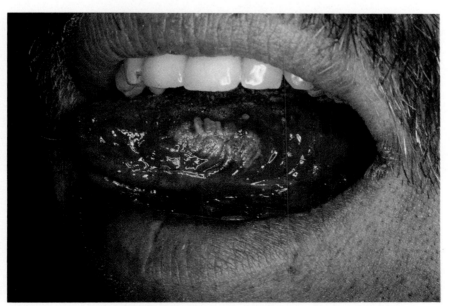

Figure 3.2 Angular cheilitis and hyperplastic candidiasis of the tongue, in this case mimicking "hairy leukoplakia". This 38 year old bisexual business executive was not aware that he was HIV positive and it was this finding that prompted HIV testing.

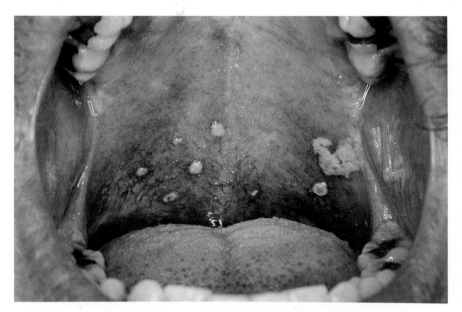

Figure 3.3   Pseudomembranous form of candidiasis in a 34 year old AIDS patient.

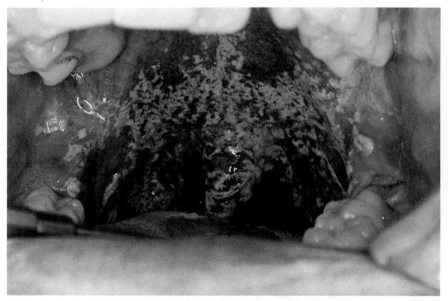

Figure 3.4   Florid candidiasis in an AIDS patient. Complaints include pain, bad breath, and altered taste.

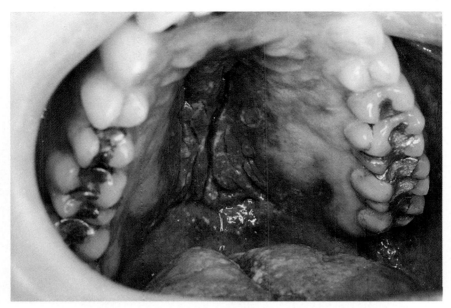

Figure 3.5   Atrophic (erythematous) form of candidiasis with minimal white-appearing surface colonies associated with AIDS. Palatal pain prompted this office visit.

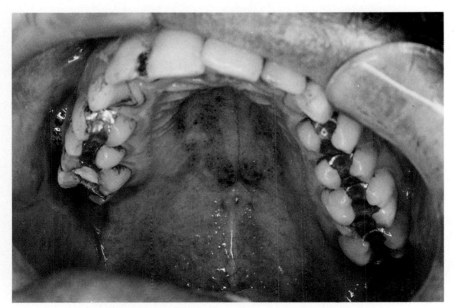

Figure 3.6   The atrophic form of candidal infection resembling telangiectatic lesions of the palate.

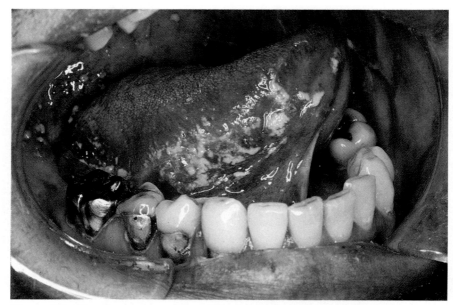

Figure 3.7 Pseudomembranous candidiasis in a 26 year old patient with ARC.

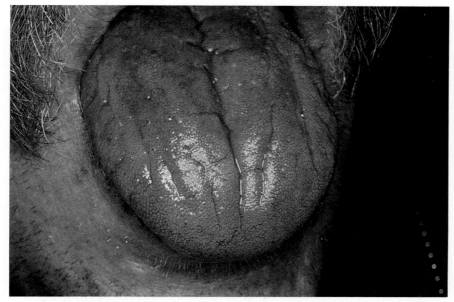

Figure 3.8 This AIDS patient sought consultation because of a severe burning sensation of the tongue associated with the atrophic form of candidiasis. Antifungal treatment reversed the signs and symptoms.

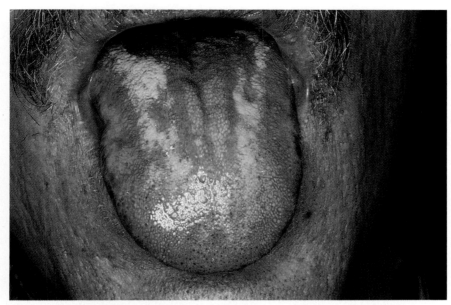

Figure 3.9   Lingual candidiasis causing an abnormal pattern of filiform papillae and surface fungal colonies. Signs were returned to normal following antifungal medication, and further scrapings tested negative.

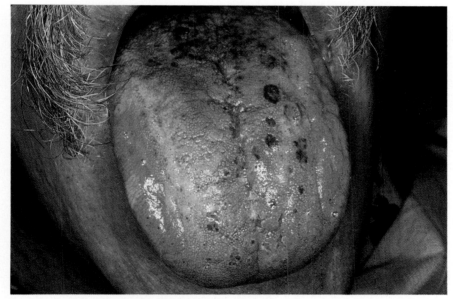

Figure 3.10   Candidal tongue lesions that at first were thought to be possible manifestations of a blood dyscrasia or a peculiar form of glossitis migrans.

Laboratory Diagnosis

To confirm the clinical suspicion of candidiasis, many laboratory procedures can be used. These include the following:

1. A surface scraping placed on a microscopic slide and prepared with potassium hydroxide or a suitable stain enables visualization of spores, hyphae, and mycelia (Figure 3.11).

2. Cultures of smears from saliva or mucosal surfaces grown on a selective solid medium support fungal colony growth (Figure 3.12). This confirms fungal presence, and also allows a quantitation as well as speciation. Quantitation is useful for determining the concentration of organisms, which is helpful in following the effectiveness of treatment, and may even be helpful in differentiating normal candida flora from pathologic overgrowth.

3. Laboratory tests for fungal speciation are based primarily on different metabolic reactions to carbohydrates. At present about 90 percent of all oral fungal infections appear to be due to *Candida albicans*. Oral infections by other candida species do not appear to have any significance, since all candidal infections respond to similar treatment and have not produced different clinical findings.

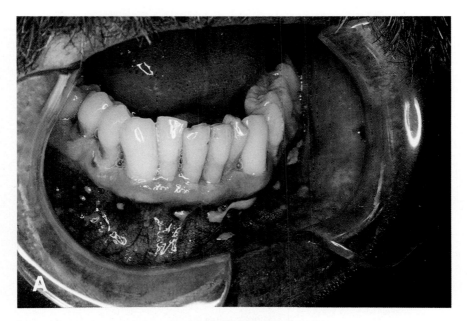

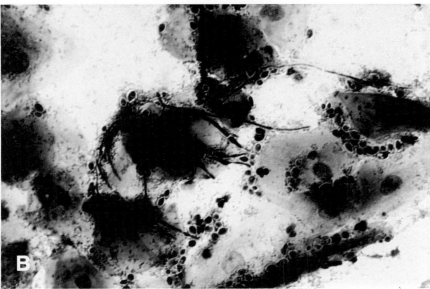

Figure 3.11   (A) Gingival and mucosal candidiasis in a 30 year old ARC patient who also had precocious periodontal disease. The mucosal lesions resembled somewhat those of a hypersensitivity reaction (erythema multiforme). (B) A gingivo-labial smear from the patient in *A* revealed hyphae, mycelia, and spores consistent with a fungal infection (Gram stain). Note the background of squamous cells. The lesions cleared with antifungal therapy.

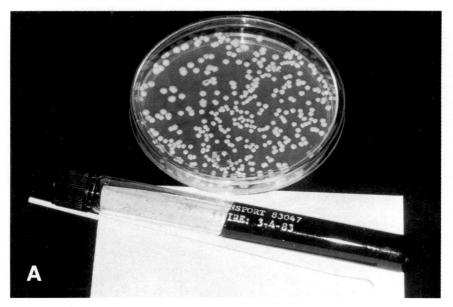

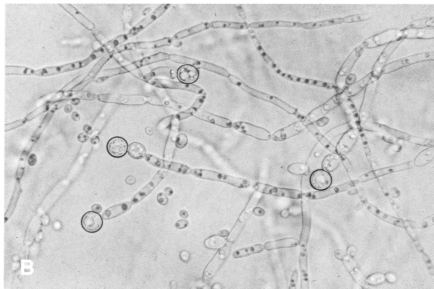

Figure 3.12 (A) A culture positive for *Candida albicans.* Note the white fungal colonies grown on Sabouraud's dextrose agar. (B) Smear of a white colony seen in *A* and observed microscopically. Note classical candida pseudomycelia and chlamyda-spores.

Biopsy

1. Biopsy specimens stained by the periodic acid Schiff method will also clearly reveal candidal organisms that may be present on or in surface epithelium (Figure 3.13). Invasion beyond surface epithelial cells has not been shown in human oral specimens.

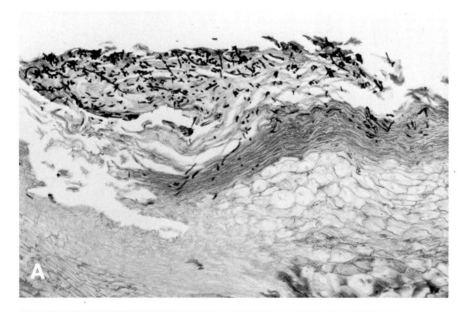

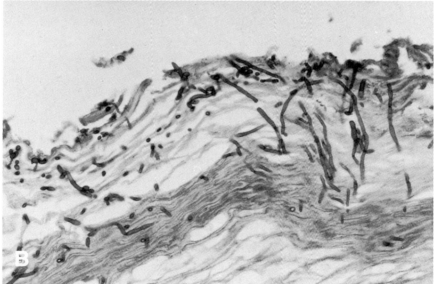

Figure 3.13   (A) Mucosal biopsy from a patient with oral candidiasis. (B) Higher power demonstrating various candidal forms growing in the superficial cell layers of the stratified squamous epithelium.

TREATMENT

Treatment of oral candidiasis is usually effective, at least until the terminal stages of HIV infection are encountered (Figures 3.14–3.17). The main problem in control is that fungal infections are usually chronic and require repeated or continual treatment. The therapeutic approach entails the use of systemic and topical antifungals, and the incorporation of antiseptic mouth rinses.

Ketoconazole (Nizoral), 200 to 400 mg with food once daily, is very effective. It is absorbed in an acid environment, and therefore ingestion with food and/or acid beverage is important to obtain optimal absorption and blood levels. In severe cases, sometimes the 400 mg dosage is required twice daily. The reasons for this may range from poor absorption to the need for greater blood/tissue concentrations. Resistance has been noted, but is uncommon. Although ketoconazole is metabolized in the liver, elevation of liver enzymes is rare, as are allergic reactions. Slightly more often patients will complain of headaches or nausea. Systemic therapy is usually intermittent and short-term, and alternately supported by topical antifungal drugs or mouth rinses. Newer systemic antifungal drugs, such as fluconazole, show evidence of even greater effectiveness. This seems to be due to better absorption (higher blood levels) and less toxicity (fewer adverse side effects).

Useful topical antifungal medications inclue nystatin and clotrimazole in forms that can be dissolved orally and then either swallowed or emptied. Nystatin can be used in the form of Mycostatin vaginal tablets, 100,000 units, dissolved orally up to five times daily. Nystatin can also be obtained in other forms: as pastilles, the effectiveness of which has not as yet been determined; and as a suspension, which some patients find difficult to hold in the mouth for long enough periods to adequately make contact and suppress the fungi. Clotrimazole can be used as 10 mg oral troches (Mycelex), dissolved up to five times daily. Another effective form of clotrimazole has been the 100 mg vaginal tablet (Gyne-Lotrimin), dissolved orally at bedtime or even twice daily. For both nystatin and clotrimazole, no rinsing or eating should take place for some time afterward so as to allow maximum exposure. Although the swallowed saliva may be effective on other segments of the gastrointestinal tract, little to none is absorbed into the blood stream, and therefore no systemic effects occur.

The mouth rinses that have been helpful include Peridex (0.12 percent chlorhexidine) and Listerine (mixture of essential oils: thymol, eucalyptol, methylsalicylate, menthol). With either rinse, patients are instructed to hold 20 cc in their mouth for up to one minute two to three times daily, then avoid rinsing for 30 to 60 minutes after emptying the contents. Since both solutions contain alcohol, some patients may experience a transient "burning" sensation. Another mouth rinse that may have some utility in fungal control is 3 percent hydrogen peroxide mixed with equal parts warm saline.

When patients are hospitalized and oral candidiasis is a complication, intravenous amphotericin B is an effective antifungal agent.

It must be remembered that candidal overgrowth is nurtured by antibiotics. Therefore, antifungal medications are often given simultaneously with antibiotics as a prophylactic measure to prevent fungal overgrowth in high risk individuals. Additionally, xerostomia occurs occasionally either as a result of idiopathic sialadenitis or from medications that reduce saliva production. In such situations the chance of developing oral candidiasis increases, and control, in addition to antifungal medication, often requires the use of a sialogogue, frequent plain water rinses, or a saliva substitute. The most common and effective sialogogue is bethanechol. Effective dosages may vary between 25 mg three times daily to 50 mg four times a day.

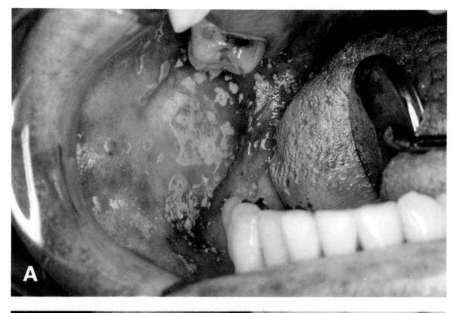

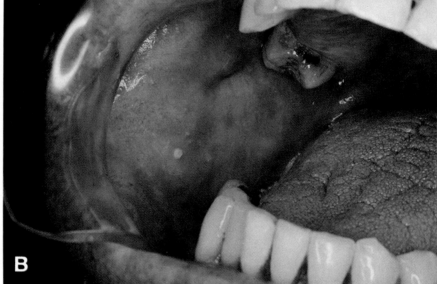

Figure 3.14   (A) A mixture of pseudomembranous and hyperplastic candidiasis in a 42 year old bisexual man. This was the initial complaint that led to the diagnosis of HIV infection. (B) Topical antifungal medication led to clearing in one week. However, the patient's immunosuppression continued to deteriorate and candidal recurrences became more frequent, more severe, and less responsive.

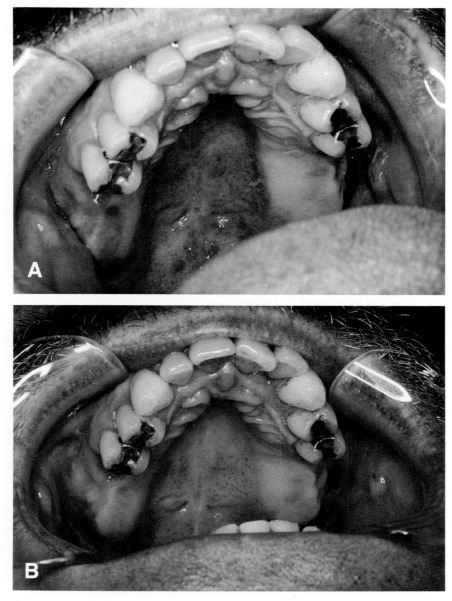

Figure 3.15   (A) Painful atrophic candidal palatal infection in an otherwise asymptomatic gay man with ARC. (B) Signs and symptoms disappeared after one week on topical antifungal medication.

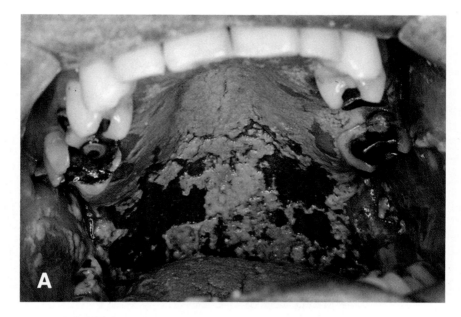

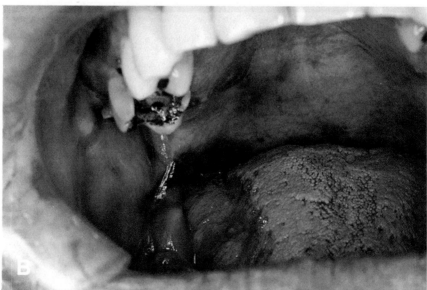

Figure 3.16 (A) Florid candidiasis in a homosexual male who did not realize he was HIV positive. This was his only complaint. (B) Systemic antifungal medication cleared the candida lesions. However, the underlying purple-red lesions were then observed, and confirmed by biopsy as Kaposi's sarcoma. He obviously had AIDS, and died 4 months later of *pneumocystis carinii* pneumonia.

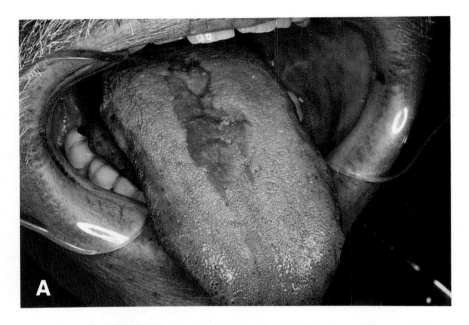

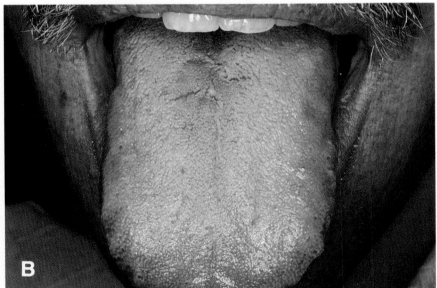

Figure 3.17 (A) This otherwise asymptomatic gay male had a painful depapillated area on his tongue dorsum. A scraping showed candidiasis and a subsequent serology revealed HIV antibodies. (B) Systemic antifungal medication reversed the signs and symptoms in one week.

REFERENCES

Epstein JB, Truelove EL, Izutzu KT. Oral candidiasis: Pathogenesis and host defense. Rev Infect Dis 1984; 6:96–106.

Klein RS, Harris CA, Small CB, et al. Oral candidiasis in high-risk patients as the initial manifestation of the acquired immunodeficiency syndrome. N Engl J Med 1984; 311:354–358.

Matthews R, Smith D, Midgley J, et al. Evidence for protective antibody. Lancet, July 1988; Vol. I.: 263–266.

Odds FC. Candida and candidosis. A review and bibliography. 2nd edition. Philadelphia: WB Saunders, 1988.

Phelan JA, Saltzman BR, Friedland GH, Klein RS. Oral findings in patients with acquired immunodeficiency syndrome. Oral Surg Oral Med Oral Pathol 1987; 64:50–56.

Rhoads JL, Wright DC, Redfield RR, Burke DS. Chronic vaginal candidiasis in women with human immunodeficiency virus infection. JAMA 1987; 257:3105–3107.

Samaranayke LP. Oral candidosis: predisposing factors and pathogenesis. In Derrick DD, ed. The 1989 dental annual. London: Wright 1989, 219–235.

Syrjanen S, Valle S-L, Antonen J, et al. Oral candidal infection as a sign of HIV infection in homosexual men. Oral Surg Oral Med Oral Pathol 1988; 65:36–40.

4

VIRAL INFECTIONS

$\mathbf{A}$t the present time there is no evidence that the AIDS virus (HIV) per se directly causes any of the oral viral infections, although HIV protein has been reported as being found in some oral epithelial cells. However, enhanced by the immunosuppression induced by HIV infection, a variety of viral infections affect the oral and paraoral regions in much greater frequency and severity than in individuals with normal immune competence. It must also be remembered that these viral infections can also be transmitted, and therefore pose a danger by close contact, particularly in others that may have immunodysregulation.

HERPES FAMILY VIRUSES

Herpes Simplex Virus

Herpes simplex virus 1 (HSV-1), and sometimes HSV-2, are rather commonly observed in HIV infected individuals, and certainly this occurs more frequently than one would expect in the general population. The main expression appears to be in the form of reactivated HSV-1 affecting the lips (herpes labialis, cold sores). In immunosuppressed individuals the lesions usually recur more frequently, they are larger, many times appear as multiple lesions, and persist longer (Fig. 4.1). In some cases the lip lesions become contiguous with the adjacent skin and they continue to expand in size and may respond poorly to treatment (Figs. 4.2 and 4.3). If mucocutaneous herpes are progressive and persist more than one month in a HIV-positive person, this condition then meets the Centers for Disease Control definition of AIDS.

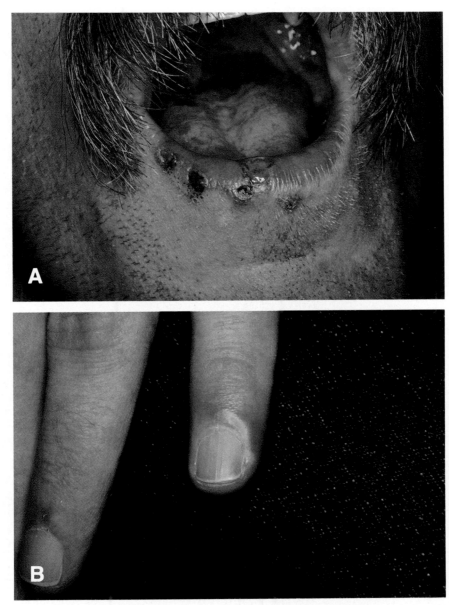

Figure 4.1 (A) This 28 year old homosexual male, who in the past had only occasional attacks of "cold sores," started manifesting multiple herpes labialis lesions that would continually recur. He was HIV positive and was afflicted with other opportunistic infections. (B) He was a nail biter and infected his nail beds with herpes simplex virus (herpetic whitlow).

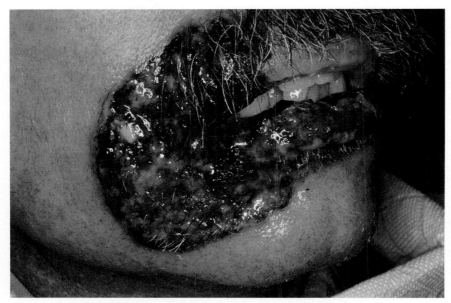

Figure 4.2 This patient had herpes labialis that was not self-limiting, and the infection spread to the adjacent skin. HSV infections that are progressive and persist for more than one month meet the CDC definition of AIDS in HIV-positive persons.

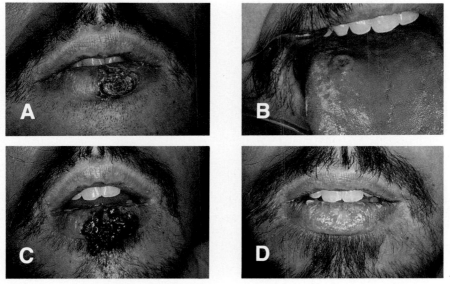

Figure 4.3 This HIV-positive homosexual male started developing cold sores that were much more severe and persisted for longer periods of time than he previously experienced. (A) This herpetic lip lesion had persisted for three weeks. (B) He also developed a lesion on the right dorsal tongue which is typical for recurrent intraoral herpetic lesions in immunocompromised patients. It is commonly found in kidney transplant patients. (C) At four weeks the lip lesion continued to extend and required treatment with acyclovir (1200 mg daily). (D) After ten days of treatment the lesion was brought under complete control.

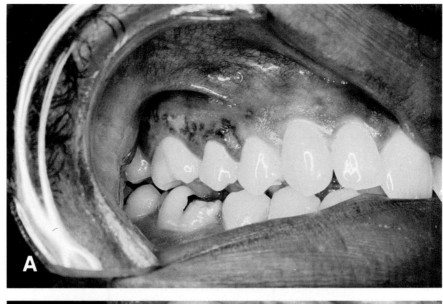

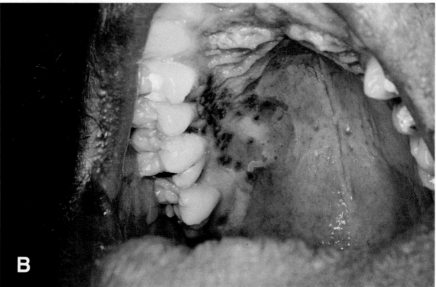

Figure 4.4 Recurrent intraoral herpetic lesions seen commonly in non-immunocompromised patients, but also found in immunocompromised patients and more frequently. (A) Recurrent HSV of gingiva. (B) Recurrent HSV of palate.

Recurrent intra-oral HSV infection can occur in the classical form of shallow, irregular ulcerations, that often have a tendency to coalesce, afflicting keratinized squamous epithelium of the hard palate, gingivae, and tongue dorsum (Fig. 4.4). Additionally and similar to infection in other immunocompromised states, recurrent intra-oral HSV can occur on any mucosal surface, and is not "restricted" to keratinized epithelia (Figs. 4.5 and 4.6). In these instances, the lesions are usually irregular in shape, vary in size if multiple, and are covered by pseudomembranes. These ulcerative lesions may or may not be associated with erythema. The ulcerations are usually quite painful and, if not treated, they can be progressive or at least persist for extended periods of time.

The clinical diagnosis can be confused with toxic and allergic reactions, or manifestations of bacterial infections. The diagnosis can be confirmed by cytologic scrapings (pseudogiant cells, demonstrating atypical multinucleation from abnormal nuclear protein production), culture techniques (cytopathologic effects caused by giant cell formation of infected cells in tissue culture if the inoculum contains HSV), or smears reacted with HSV-specific monoclonal antibodies.

When there is evidence that a patient can still mount an antibody defense, management can be instituted utilizing empirical approaches. However, specific therapy is accomplished primarily by using acyclovir (Zovirax). Since acyclovir is poorly absorbed, large doses (1 to 4 grams) are required. Acyclovir prevents viral replication by interfering with DNA polymerase when the acyclovir is phosphorylated. Phosphorylation occurs in the presence of the viral enzyme, thymidine kinase. Toxic reactions are rare; however, in a small percentage of patients a resistance, which can be temporary, is developed. Prophylactic regimens are still in trial-and-error stages. Recurrences are unpredictable.

It is of interest that a new human herpes virus (HHV-6) has been shown to facilitate infection of host cells in vitro. Therefore, evidence may be mounting that HSV infections by certain types may be important cofactors in host susceptibility.

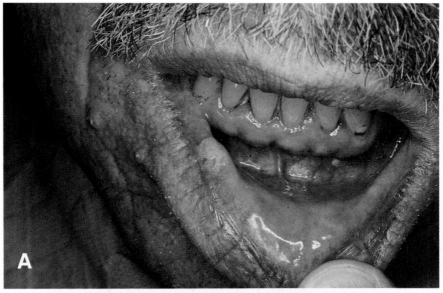

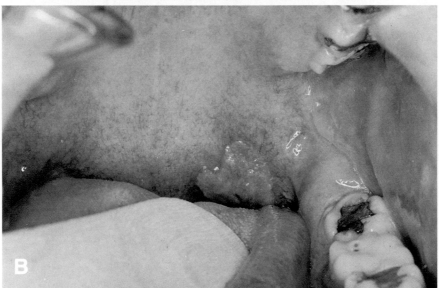

Figure 4.5   Recurrent intraoral herpes in immunocompromised patients can occur in any mucosal site. They appear typically as pseudomembraned-covered mucosal erosions of irregular sizes and shapes. (A) Reccurent HSV of labial mucosa. (B) Recurrent HSV of soft palate.

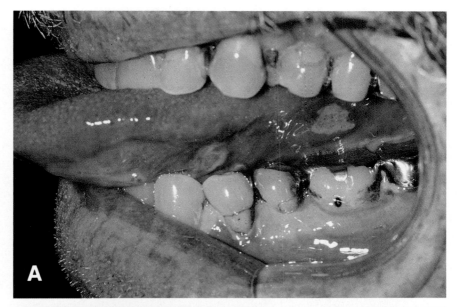

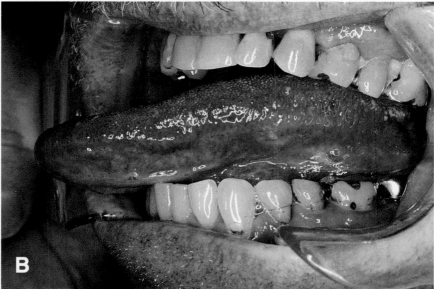

Figure 4.6   Recurrent HSV usually responds quite well to acyclovir in daily dosages exceeding 1 gram. This treatment is usually effective until the terminal stages of AIDS. (A) Increasingly painful HSV lesions of the tongue that persisted over 2 weeks in a 32 year old HIV-positive man. (B) Signs and symptoms rapidly disappeared after four days of systemic acyclovir (1200 milligrams daily).

Epstein-Barr Virus and Hairy Leukoplakia

Epstein-Barr virus (EBV) infection may be a cofactor in the occurrence of non-Hodgkin's lymphoma (Chapter 6), as well as serve the role of promoter for other oral lesions. Of greatest importance is the association of EBV and the presence of oral "hairy leukoplakia" (HL). HL describes white-appearing lesions that almost always occur unilaterally or bilaterally on the lateral borders of the tongue (Figs. 4.7–4.16). HL frequently appears as hair-like projections and/or corrugations, but it may also have a plaque-like appearance. Thus, the name "hairy leukoplakia." Uncommonly HL will appear on other oral sites, such as the buccal mucosa, oropharynx, and mouth floor. There is no evidence that this is similar to hyperkeratotic leukoplakia that has premalignant connotations.

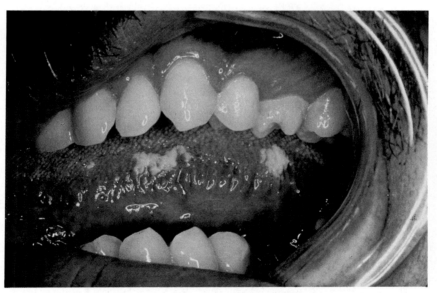

Figure 4.7   Limited hairy leukoplakia in an asymptomatic HIV-positive homosexual male.

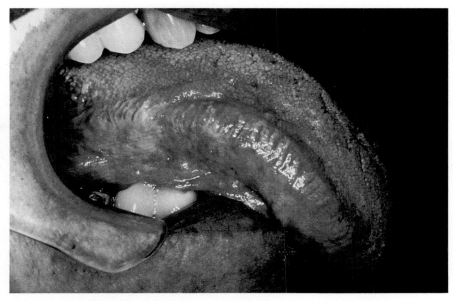

Figure 4.8   Limited asymptomatic hairy leukoplakia in a 30 year old homosexual male. He was otherwise in apparent good health; but this was the first sign of HIV infection.

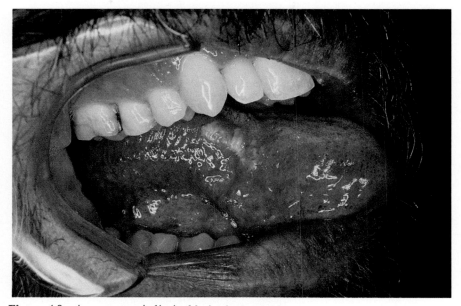

Figure 4.9   Asymptomatic limited hairy leukoplakia.

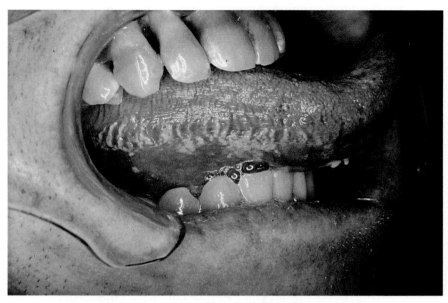

Figure 4.10 A more typical appearance of hairy leukoplakia, demonstrating the corrugated and hair-like appearance that prompted the name.

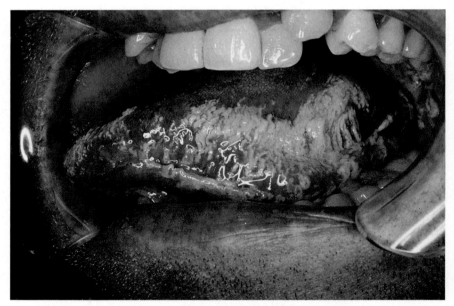

Figure 4.11 A more extensive hairy leukoplakia in a 30 year old homosexual male. He also had oropharyngeal candidiasis; however, the oral candidiasis responded to anti-fungal treatment, while the hairy leukoplakia lesion remained. It was essentially asymptomatic.

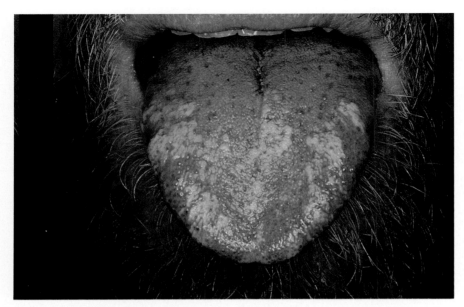

Figure 4.12   The hairy leukoplakia in this 27 year old homosexual extended onto the tongue dorsum. Except for a mild chronic candidiasis, the patient was without any other signs or symptoms. Six months later he developed *Pneumocystis carinii* pneumonia.

Microscopically HL appears as an epithelial hyperplasia with a parakeratotic surface and vacuolated cells often referred to as koilocytes (cells suggestive of viral infection) (Fig. 4.17). The presence of EBV in these vacuolated cells has been confirmed by electron microscopy and DNA probes. Sometimes non-HL lesions can have similar clinical, and even microscopic appearances. Thus, ultimate confirmation is the demonstration of EBV. Connective tissue inflammation may vary from moderate white cell infiltrates to the appearance of a non-inflammatory lesion.

The cause of HL is unknown. Whether EBV is a cause or result is as yet not clear. HL can occur in all-HIV infected groups, although it is by far more common in homosexual and bisexual men. Of utmost importance is the significance that HL indicates HIV infection and is highly predictive for the development of AIDS, in most individuals probably within 3 years.

Treatment is elective. These lesions are usually asymptomatic, but chronic. They are treated only if they are bothersome in some way to the patient, or by coincidence when another disease is the target of treatment. HL may disappear following high doses of acyclovir, azidothymidine (zidovudine), which interrupts viral replication, topical Retin-A solution, and sulfa-type antibiotics given for controlling pneumocystis pneumonia. HL usually recurs when treatment is modified or discontinued. In any event, HL augurs for a poor prognosis and is most definitely a sign of HIV infection.

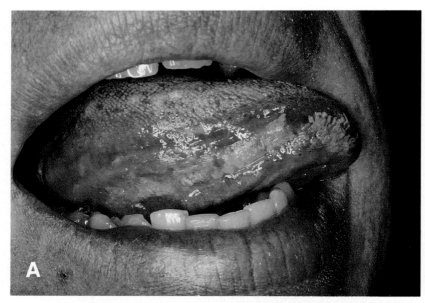

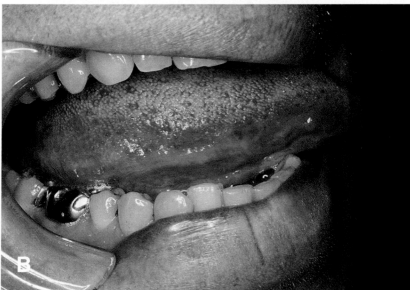

Figure 4.13   Treatment is non-specific and elective. (A) Mildly symptomatic hairy leukoplakia. The patient also had pneumocystis pneumonia and was put on azidothymidine (AZT). (B) After one month on daily AZT, and without any other forms of management, the hairy leukoplakia essentially disappeared clinically.

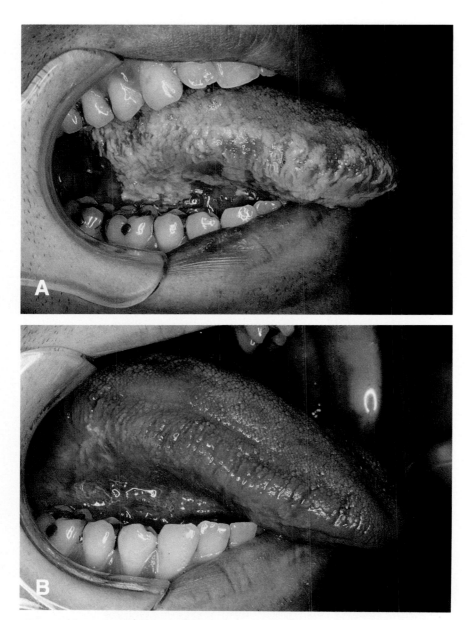

Figure 4.14   Most hairy leukoplakias will go into clinical remission on large doses of acyclovir. (A) Pre-treatment appearance. (B) Appearance following 2 grams of daily acyclovir for 2 weeks. When the acyclovir was discontinued, the lesion slowly returned to the same site and extent.

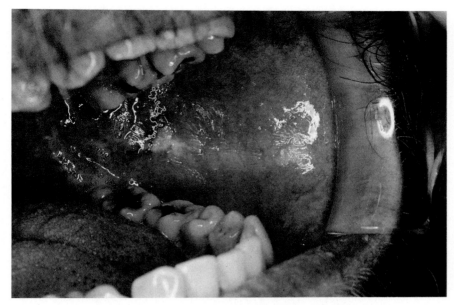

Figure 4.15   Hairy leukoplakia occasionally will occur on sites other than the lateral borders of the tongue. This 32 year old HIV-positive homosexual male had biopsy-proven hairy leukoplakia on the buccal mucosa as well as the tongue.

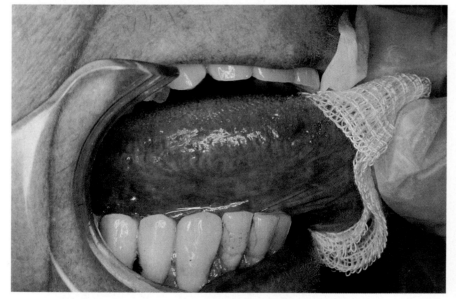

Figure 4.16   Many lesions may resemble hairy leukoplakia. Because of the significance regarding HIV infection implied by hairy leukoplakia, clinical suspicion must be confirmed. This patient who was concerned about being immunocompromised had biopsy-proven lichen planus. A subsequent serology showed her to be HIV negative.

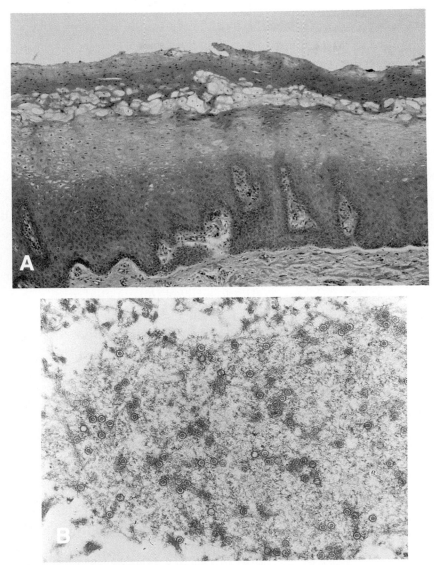

Figure 4.17 Histopathology of hairy leukoplakia is used to confirm the clinical impression. (A) Classical appearance of hairy leukoplakia, demonstrating epithelial hyperplasia, little or no connective tissue inflammation, a pseudo-keratin surface layer, and multiple vacuolated cells associated with Epstein-Barr virus infection. The vacuolated cells have been referred to as koilocytes, implying viral infection. (B) An electron microscopic photomicrograph of part of a nucleus of a vacuolated cell, demonstrating Epstein-Barr viruses interspersed in the nuclear protein.

Varicella Virus (Zoster, Shingles)

In the immunocompromised patient, the risk exists for reactivation of latent chicken pox virus. When this occurs, the disease takes the form of varicella zoster, more commonly referred to as herpes zoster or shingles (Fig. 4.18). The epithelial vesicles formed by the virus eventually burst and scab, and have a classical unilateral distribution. They are painful as well as pruritic. While the lesions are almost always self-limiting, the most bothersome part of the infection is the post-zoster neuropathy, with associated pain that is often quite disabling. Treatment is empirical, utilizing acyclovir, analgetics, and tricyclic/mood-altering medications. Recurrences, even in the immunocompromised group, are uncommon. When varicella zoster occurs in the HIV-infected patient, the prognosis for developing AIDS is grave, and expiring in a relatively short period of time from an opportunistic infection is likely.

Cytomegalovirus

Cytomegalovirus (CMV) antibodies are found in over 50 percent of the normal population indicating the commonality of human exposure to this virus. CMV can cause a mononucleosis-like illness. In HIV-infected individuals, antibodies to CMV are almost always found, and in a considerable number, the virus can actually be cultivated. In immunocompromised patients, CMV can cause retinitis, leukopenia, hepatitis, gastrointestinal ulcerations, and pneumonitis. Oral muco sal lesions induced by CMV are rarely recognized or reported and have not reproducibly been documented. However, CMV may serve as a cofactor in the development of other mouth conditions. For example, since CMV has a predilection for major salivary glands, one speculation concerns the possibility of CMV induced major salivary gland inflammation which may cause facial swelling, or the alteration of saliva production, possibly accounting for the somewhat common complaint of xerostomia (Chapter 7).

Human Papillomavirus

There are numerous types of the human papillomaviruses (HPV), numbering over 55. These viruses are so commonly found, their relationship to various diseases is often difficult to document, that is, causal, cofactor, or passenger. One condition of known cause-and-effect relationship is that related to condyloma acuminata (venereal warts). These warts can occur on any mucosal surface, and can resemble small fibromas, squamous papillomas, or verrucae (Figs. 4.19–4.25). Most patients who have oral condyloma will often have genital or anal warts also. Although having venereal warts doesn't necessarily mean that a person is HIV infected, it is associated with a lifestyle and behavior that put a patient at risk to being exposed to the AIDS virus. In a considerable number of such patients, the oral warts have been the first sign that have prompted HIV testing.

The diagnosis is made on the basis of history, clinical appearance, and biopsy. Treatment is often complex, since control depends upon adequate surgical removal of the oral warts, concomitant therapy if there are genito-anal warts, treating partners who may already be infected, and counseling regarding future behavior and protection/prevention barrier techniques. Obviously these lesions are infectious both to spread within the host as well as to partners.

The roles of HPV relative to other oral lesions, for example leukoplakias and carcinomas, continue to be investigated.

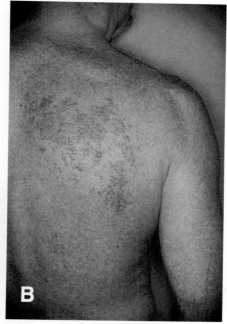
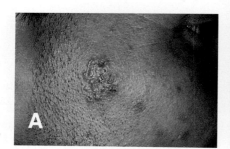

Figure 4.18   Varicella zoster (shingles) in a 42 year old homosexual male with AIDS. This patient in addition to having vesicles unilaterally on the face (A) and back (B), also had Kaposi's sarcoma of the palate, chronic diarrhea, and an increasing number of allergies.

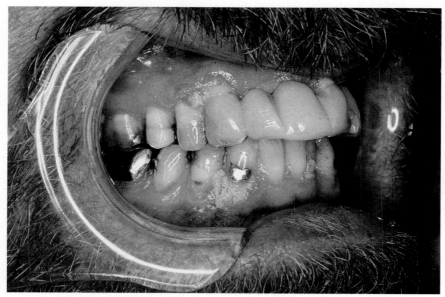

Figure 4.19   Multiple venereal warts (condyloma acuminata) of the gingiva in this 34 year old HIV-positive homosexual man.

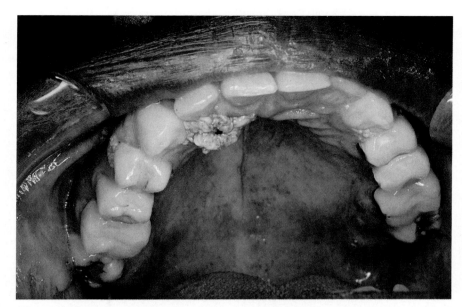

Figure 4.20   A large venereal wart in a homosexual male, who also has venereal warts on the genitalia.

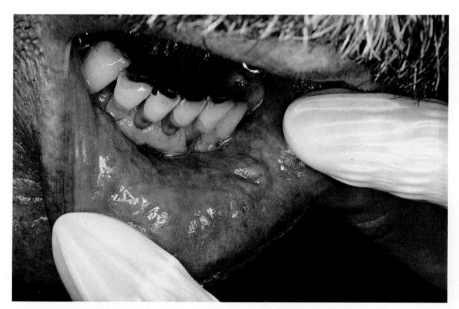

Figure 4.21   Venereal wart of the lower lip in a sexually active HIV-positive homosexual man.

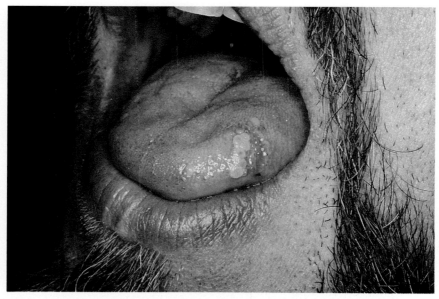

Figure 4.22   Venereal wart of the tongue that was mildly bothersome to the patient. This HIV-positive man also had anal condylomata.

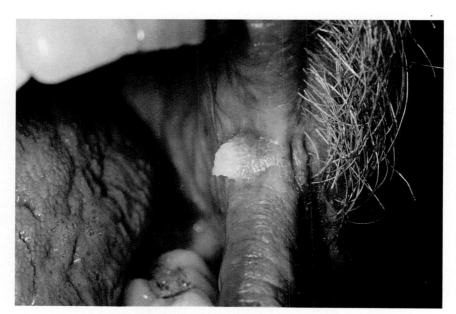

Figure 4.23   A large symptomatic venereal wart of the left commissure in this HIV-positive homosexual male.

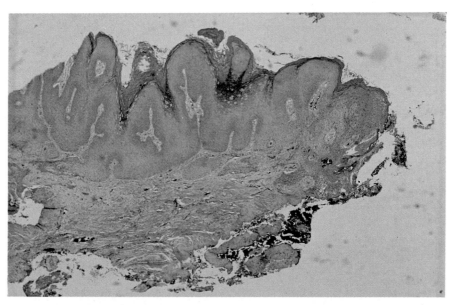

Figure 4.24   Classical histologic presentation of a venereal wart, demonstrating irregular epithelial hyperplasia, hyperkeratosis, and vacuolated epithelial cells that are infected with various types of human papillomavirus.

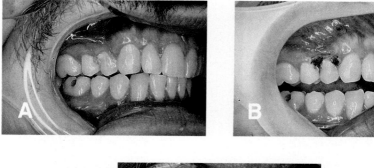

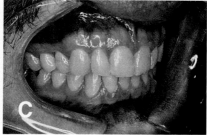

Figure 4.25   Treatment of condylomata involves excision of the warts, along with simultaneous control of any genital or anal warts, and care of partners. Otherwise the infection will continually recur. (A) Venereal warts involving the upper right first bicuspid gingiva. (B) Excision and cauterization to remove clinical lesion and associated virus. (C) Follow-up at one week indicating at least temporary control.

REFERENCES

Herpes Simplex

Cohen SG, Greenberg MS. Chronic oral herpes simplex virus infection in immunocompromised patients. Oral Surg Oral Med Oral Pathol 1985; 59:465–471.

Glatt AE, Chirgwin K, Landesman SH. Current concepts. Treatment of infections associated with human immunodeficiency virus. N Engl J Med 1988; 318:1439–1448.

Lafferty WE, Coombs RW, Benedetti J, et al. Recurrences after oral and genital herpes simplex infection. Influence of site of infection and viral type. N Engl J Med 1987; 316:1444–1449.

Molinari JA, Merchant VA. Herpesviruses. Manifestations and transmissions. Calif Dent Assoc J 1989; 17:24–31.

Perma JJ, Eskinazi DP. Treatment of oro-facial herpes simplex infections with acyclovir: a review. Oral Surg Oral Med Oral Pathol 1988; 65:889–892.

Raborn GW, McGaw WJ, Grace M, et al. Oral acyclovir and herpes labialis: a randomized, double-blind, placebo-controlled study. JADA 1987; 115:38–42.

Raymond CA. Evidence mounts that other infections may trigger AIDS virus replication. JAMA 1987; 257:2875.

Shaw M, King M, Best JM, et al. Failure of acyclovir cream on treatment of recurrent herpes labialis. Brit Med J 1985; 291:7–9.

Hairy Leukoplakia

Ficarra G, Barone R, Gaglioti D, Milo D, et al. Oral hairy leukoplakia among HIV-positive intravenous drug abusers: a clinicopathologic and ultrastructural study. Oral Surg Oral Med Oral Pathol 1988; 65:421–426.

Green TL, Greenspan JS, Greenspan D, De Souza YG. Oral lesions mimicking hairy leukoplakia: a diagnostic dilemma. Oral Surg Oral Med Oral Pathol 1989; 67:442–426.

Greenspan D, Greenspan JS, Hearst NG, et al. Relation of oral hairy leukoplakia to infection with the human immunodeficiency virus and the risk of developing AIDS. J Infect Dis 1987; 155:475–481.

Greenspan JS, Greenspan D. Oral hairy leukoplakia: diagnosis and management. oral Surg Oral Med Oral Pathol 1989; 67:396–403.

Greenspan JS, Greenspan D, Lennette ET, et al. Replication of Epstein-Bar virus within the epithelial cells of oral "hairy" leukoplakia, an AIDS-associated lesion. N Engl J Med 1985; 313:1564–1571.

Kanas RJ, Abrams AM, Jensen JL, et al. Oral hairy leukoplakia: ultrastructural observations. Oral Surg Oral Med Oral Pathol 1988; 65:333–338.

Phelan JA, Klein RS. Resolution of oral hairy leukoplakia during treatment with azidothymidine. Oral Surg Oral Med Oral Pathol 1988; 65:717–720.

Rindum JL, Schiodt M, Pindborg JJ, Scheibel E. Oral hairy leukoplakia in three hemophiliacs with human immunodeficiency virus infection. Oral Surg Oral Med Oral Pathol 1987; 63:437–440.

Schiodt M, Greenspan D, Daniels TE, Greenspan JS. Clinical and histologic spectrum of oral hairy leukoplakia. Oral Surg Oral Med Oral Pathol 1987; 64:716–720.

Sciubba J, Brandsma J, Schwartz M, Barrezveta N. Hairy leukoplakia: an AIDS-associated opportunistic infection. Oral Surg Oral Med Oral Pathol 1989; 67:404–410.

Cytomegalovirus

Kanas RJ, Jensen JJ, Abrams AM, Wuerker RB. Oral mucosal cytomegalovirus as a manifestation of the acquired immune deficiency syndrome. Oral Surg Oral Med Oral Pathol 1987; 64:183–189.

Marder M, Barr CE, Mandel ID. Cytomegalovirus presence and salivary composition in acquired immunodeficiency syndrome. Oral Surg Oral Med Oral Pathol 1985; 60:372–376.

Zoster

Melbye M, Goedert JJ, Grossman RJ, et al. Risk of AIDS after herpes zoster. Lancet 1987; iii:728–731.

Weller TH. Varicella and herpes zoster. Changing concepts of the natural history, control and importance of a not-so-benign virus. N Engl J Med 1983; 309:1434–1438.

Human Papillomaviruses

Anneroth G, Anniko M, Romander H. Oral condyloma acuminatum. A light and electron microscopic study. Int J Oral Surg 1982; 11:260–264.

Barrasso R, DeBrux J, Croissant O, Orth G. High prevalence of papillomavirus-associated penile intraepithelial neoplasia in sexual partners of women with cervical intraepithelial neoplasia. N Engl J Med 1987; 317:916–923.

Boon ME, Schneider A, Hogewoning CJA, et al. Penile studies and heterosexual partners. Cancer 1988; 61:1652–1659.

Eversole LR, Laipis PJ. Oral squamous papillomas: detection of HPV DNA by in situ hybridization. Oral Surg Oral Med Oral Pathol 1988; 65:545–550.

Green TL, Eversole LR, Leider AS. Oral and labial verruca vulgaris: clinical, histologic and immunohistochemical evaluation. Oral Surg Oral Med Oral Pathol 1986; 62:410–416.

Saito K, Saito A, Fu YS, et al. Topographic study of cervical condyloma and intraepithelial neoplasia. Cancer 1987; 59:2064–2070.

Scully C, Cox MF, Prime SS, Maitland NJ. Papillomaviruses: the current status in relation to oral disease. Oral Surg Oral Med Oral Pathol 1988; 65:526–532.

5 BACTERIAL INFECTIONS

HIV-Associated Gingivitis and Periodontosis

Some years ago it became evident that unusual gingival and periodontal lesions were, with unexpected frequency, afflicting young homosexual men who were AIDS-virus infected. While a frequency figure for HIV-associated gingival (HIV-G) and periodontal (HIV-P) diseases has not yet been established by population studies of high risk groups, the more-than-expected frequency of HIV-G and HIV-P is well recognized and a reality.

Clinical characteristics include the following: (1) a gingivitis that can be manifested by necrotic ulcerative lesions and/or erythema; (2) discomfort and pain; (3) alveolar bone necrosis; and (4) rapid and progressive gingival recession and bone resorption (Figures 5.1 to 5.6). The involvement of periodontal structures creates an opportunity for early detection in those who are unaware of their HIV status; but it also raises a difficult problem in management. Concerns involve operator risks, the time and costs involved in treatment, the unpredictability of response, and the recurrence or progression of disease.

Relative to etiology, most studies are directed toward oral and subgingival microbial flora. There is a firm indication of oral flora changes; for example, an increase in subgingival gram-negative anaerobes and the presence of *Candida* species. There are also indications that alterations of salivary components, such as antimicrobial enzymes and immunoglobulins (antibodies) may play a role in flora and plaque control. In any event, HIV-G and HIV-P appear to be correlated with overall progressive host immunosuppression. Poor oral hygiene and dental neglect unquestionably complicate the problem.

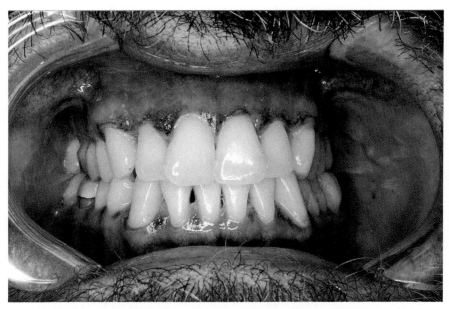

Figure 5.1   Speckled, telangiectatic-like asymptomatic gingivitis was one of the first signs of HIV infection. Although this patient was candida positive, the gingival lesions remained after antifungal treatment and a subsequent negative culture. The gingivitis was also nonresponsive to antibiotics. Blood counts were normal, as were platelets. A biopsy revealed a non-specific "mucositis."

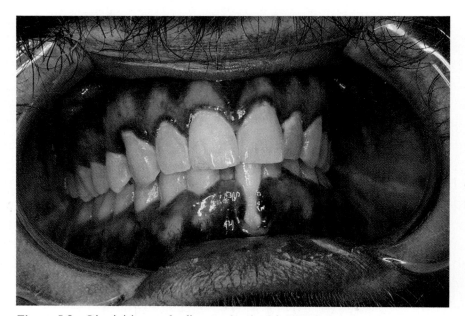

Figure 5.2   Gingivitis was the first marker in this HIV-infected patient. Note the severe gingival clefting involving the lower central incisor.

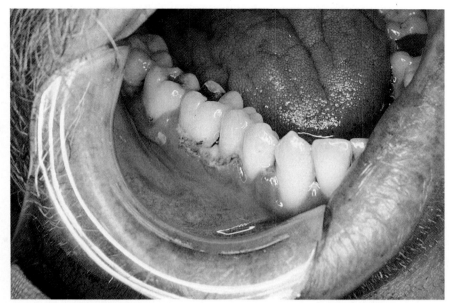

Figure 5.3   Commonly seen subacute necrotizing ulcerative gingivitis in a 32 year old HIV-positive patient. It is often progressive and requires aggressive treatment.

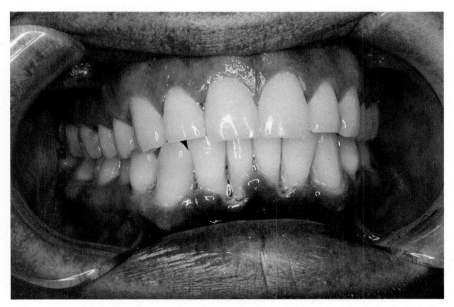

Figure 5.4   Chronic painful necrotizing, ulcerative gingivitis and periodontal disease in an otherwise asymptomatic HIV-infected 30 year old patient.

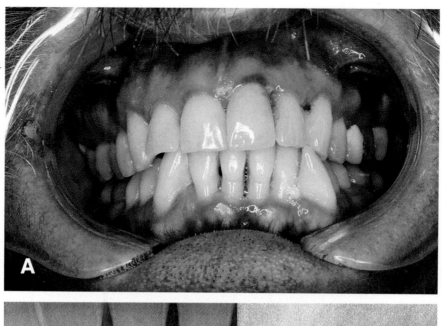

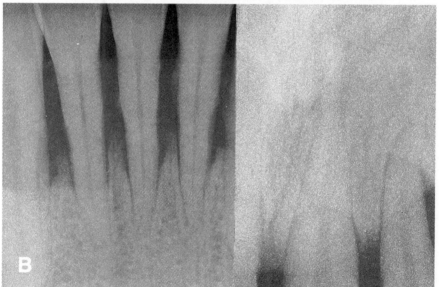

Figure 5.5   (A) Progressive gingival recession and alveolar bone resorption in an AIDS patient. Note vascular-like lesion associated with the marginal gingiva of the upper left central incisor. A biopsy of the maxillary lesion proved to be Kaposi's sarcoma and the first sign of AIDS. (B) Note radiographic evidence of loss of bone.

Bacterial Infections **59**

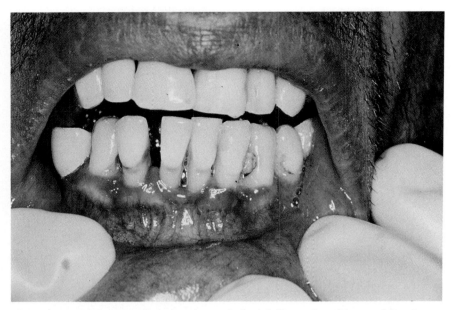

Figure 5.6 Advanced and progressive periodontal disease in a 34 year old male.

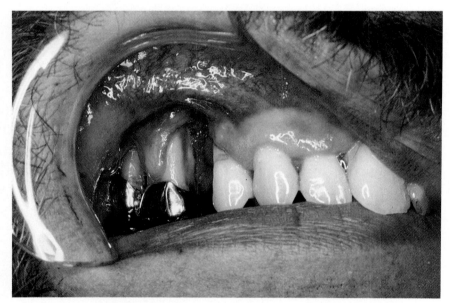

Figure 5.7 Advanced bone loss in a 29 year old patient with AIDS-related complex. Aggressive office and home care, including the use of antibiotics, was not able to control this progressive infection.

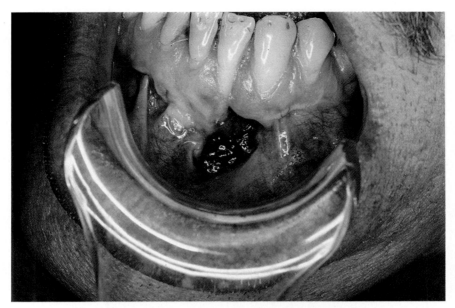

Figure 5.8 An area of mucosal and bone necrosis in this HIV-infected patient. There was no evident cause, and response to management regimes was slow.

Treatment is directed toward both office and home care (Figures 5.7 to 5.10). This involves maintaining optimal general health and nutrition, office scaling and curettage (often combined with povidone-iodine irrigations), antibiotics if necessary to control oral pathogens (metronidazole or penicillin/penicillin alternates), and fungal control if indicated. Also recommended is appropriate home care with usual, but intensive, oral hygiene approaches enhanced by daily mouth rinses, such as 0.12 percent chlorhexadine. Outcomes are variable. Unquestionably, compliance often is a problem because of attitudes, costs, and other coincidental acute complications of HIV infection.

Non-Oral Flora Opportunists

Other non-periodontal, non-dental bacterial oral infections have been reported. Some of these infections have been related to overgrowth of microorganisms that have access to the mouth, but are not a usual component of the oral flora (Figures 5.11 and 5.12). Thus, opportunistic bacteria not usually associated with oral pathology possess the capability of inducing oral mucosal signs and symptoms in the immunocompromised host.

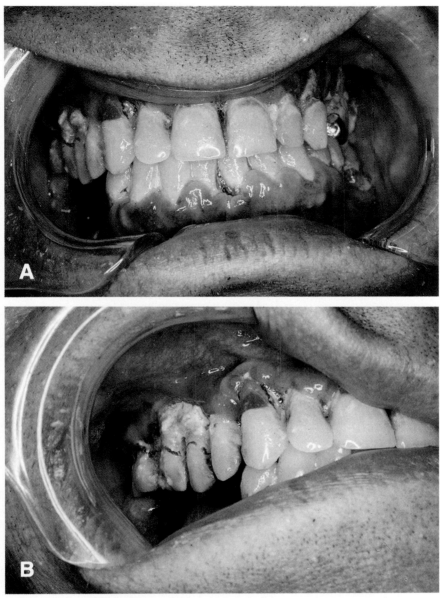

Figure 5.9 (A) This 30 year old HIV-positive drug abuser with extremely poor hygiene had progressive periodontal disease. (B) Note the osteonecrosis involving the upper right posterior quadrant. Temporary control was achieved by curettage, home care compliance, antibiotics, and a disinfectant mouth rinse.

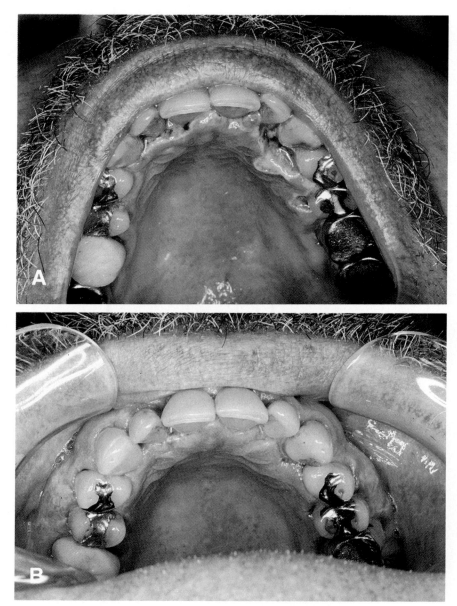

Figure 5.10 (A) Acute necrotizing ulcerative gingivitis in a 36 year old AIDS patient. T4-lymphocytes approximated 200 cells/mm³ blood. (B) Ten days of penicillin V (1500 mg daily) and peroxide–saline mouth rinses induced healing.

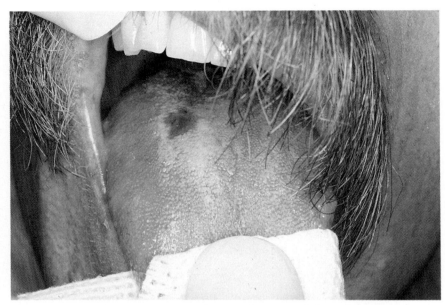

Figure 5.11 *Escherichia coli* infection causing a painful, erythematous, erosive lesion of the tongue dorsum. The diagnosis was established by culture and response to antibiotic therapy.

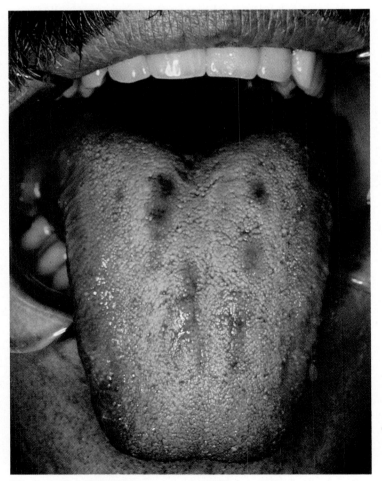

Figure 5.12 *Klebsiella pneumoniae* infection of the tongue causing painful, erythematous lesions that responded to antibiotic therapy. The diagnosis was suspected from culture results.

REFERENCES

Grassi M, Williams CA, Winkler JR, Murray PA. Management of HIV-associated periodontal diseases. Chapter 9, in Robertson PR, Greenspan JS (eds), Oral manifestations of AIDS. Littleton, Mass. PSG Publishing Co, 1988; pp 119-130.

Seymour GJ. Possible mechanisms involved in immunoregulation of chronic inflammatory periodontal disease. J Dent Res, 1987; 66:2-9.

Silverman S Jr. AIDS update: oral findings, diagnosis, and precautions. J Am Dent Assoc 1987; 115:559-563.

Winkler JR, Murray PA. AIDS update. Periodontal disease. A potential intraoral expression of AIDS may be rapidly progressive periodontitis. Calif Dent Assoc J, 1987; 15:20-24.

Winkler JR, Grassi M, Murray PA. Clinical description and etiology of HIV-associated periodontal diseases. Chapter 5, in Robertson PR, Greenspan JS (eds), Oral manifestations of AIDS. Littleton, Mass. PSG Publishing Co, 1988; pp 49-70.

6

HIV-ASSOCIATED MALIGNANCIES

Immunocompromised hosts incur a greater risk for developing malignant neoplasms. Therefore, it is not unexpected that HIV-infected individuals are afflicted with malignancies at a rate higher than would be expected in the general population.

KAPOSI'S SARCOMA

The most frequently found malignancy in AIDS patients is Kaposi's sarcoma (KS). The diagnosis of KS in a patient less than 60 years of age meets the CDC definition for AIDS. The question as to whether KS is a true cancer is often raised. However, KS will affect major organ systems, it is most commonly multicentric, and it can be the primary cause of death. Most frequently, however, patients with KS live longer than other AIDS patients, and they usually succumb to an opportunistic infection.

KS most often occurs in homosexual HIV-infected men. In this group, KS afflicts about 25 to 30 percent. The frequency of KS in all AIDS patients approximates 15 to 20 percent. These differences in occurrence cannot be explained, since KS appears to be linked to a cellular growth factor that stimulates the proliferation of blood and lymphatic vessels and fibrous connective tissue. A definitive diagnosis can be established by biopsy (Figure 6.1).

The most frequent site of KS is the skin (Figures 6.2 and 6.3). However, in cases studied in large series, about half the patients have oral KS, and in many, the oral KS is the first or only site of occurrence. While at first KS is not bothersome or even noticed by the patient, often the disease progresses and interferes with function and comfort. Therefore, professionals involved in oral health care services incur a responsibility in diagnosis, treatment, and follow-up.

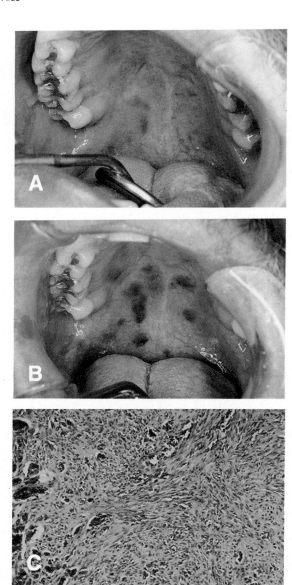

Figure 6.1   A 28 year old HIV-positive male was seen because of a slight palatal irritation. He was otherwise asymptomatic. (A) The very beginning signs of Kaposi's sarcoma were barely detectable. (B) Two months later the lesions progressed to the characteristic features of KS. The flat, vascular-appearing palatal lesions reflected "growth factor" activity, stimulating lymphatic- and vascular-endothelial and fibroblastic proliferations. (C) Biopsy of the palate confirmed KS and AIDS.

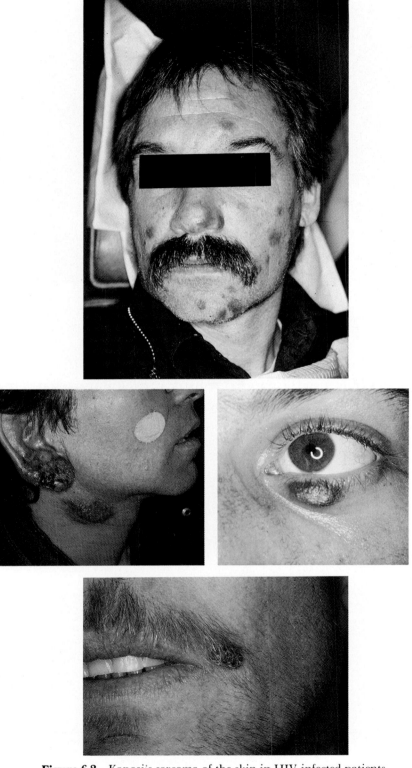

Figure 6.2   Kaposi's sarcoma of the skin in HIV-infected patients.

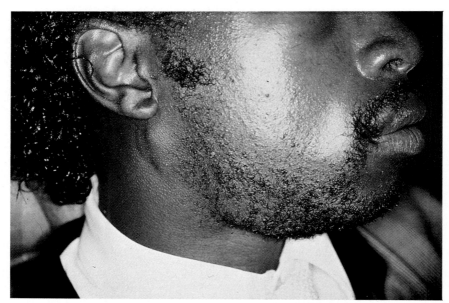

Figure 6.3 Kaposi's sarcoma involving a cervical lymph node.

KS characteristically appears as a vascular-like, bluish-red lesion (Figures 6.4 to 6.9). The areas of tumor formation are usually irregular in shape, they are most often multiple (Table 6.1), and can vary between flat discolored areas to massive proliferative tumors. In the proliferative stage, the KS can be painful, hemorrhagic, and interfere with speech, eating, and hygiene.

TABLE 6.1 University of California Study—Kaposi's Sarcoma in 134 Homosexual Males

Site		Total (%)	Single (%)	Multiple (%)
Palate		95	52	43
Gingiva		23	11	12
Oropharynx		14	13	1
Buccal		10	3	7
Tongue		10	9	1
Occurrence		*Palate*	*Gingiva*	*Others*
First sign of KS	22%	23/29	10/29	12/29
Skin simultaneously	45%	61/61	14/61	18/61
Following skin KS	33%	44/44	7/44	23/44
Total	100%	128/134	31/134	53/134

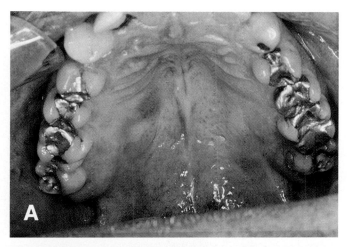

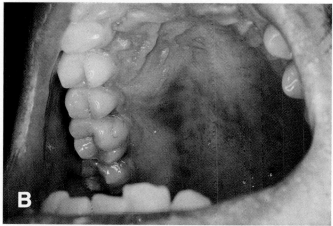

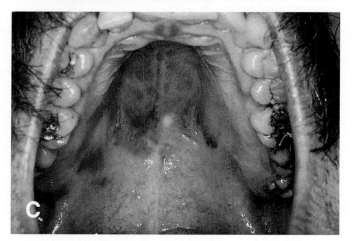

Figure 6.4   Various forms of Kaposi's sarcoma of the palate, which is the most common intraoral site. (A) Very early Kaposi's sarcoma. (B) Slightly more extensive flat KS lesions, somewhat resembling ecchymosis of trauma, hemangioma, purpura, or even a minor salivary gland tumor. (C) Extensive, flat KS, mildly symptomatic.

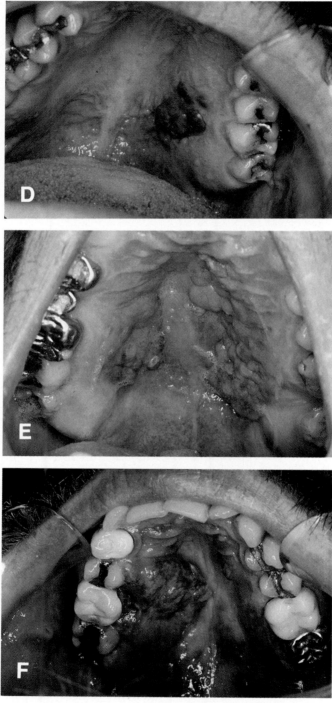

Figure 6.4 *Continued.* (D) Nodular KS. (E) Widespread nodular KS. (F) Advanced nodular KS, associated with pain, bleeding, and interfering with speech and swallowing.

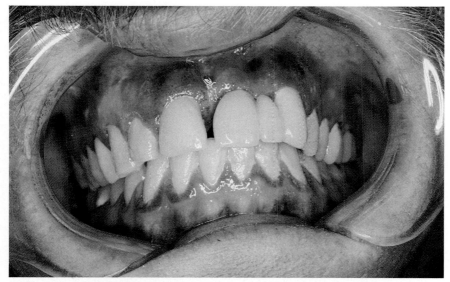

Figure 6.5 Flat, early Kaposi's sarcoma of upper gingiva. Note erythema of mandibular marginal gingiva, which is a non-KS gingivitis.

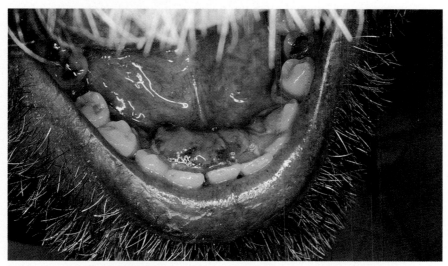

Figure 6.6 Nodular Kaposi's sarcoma involving the lower lingual gingiva.

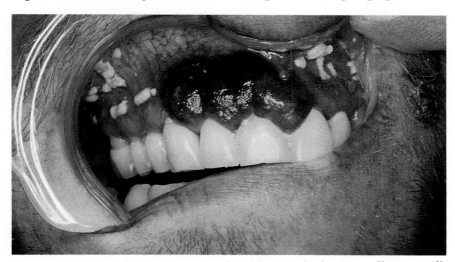

Figure 6.7 Advanced Kaposi's sarcoma involving the gingiva. Note adjacent candidal lesions.

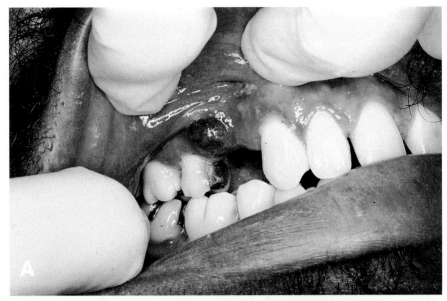

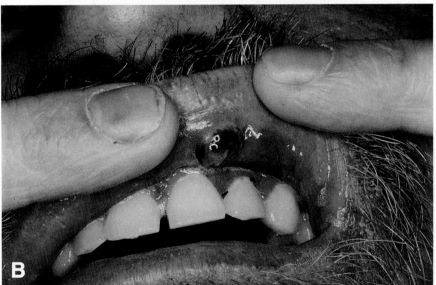

Figure 6.8 (A) Kaposi's sarcoma of the gingiva resembling a hemangioma or blood-filled parulis. (B) Kaposi's sarcoma of the labial mucosa resembling a hemangioma or a blood-filled pseudocyst.

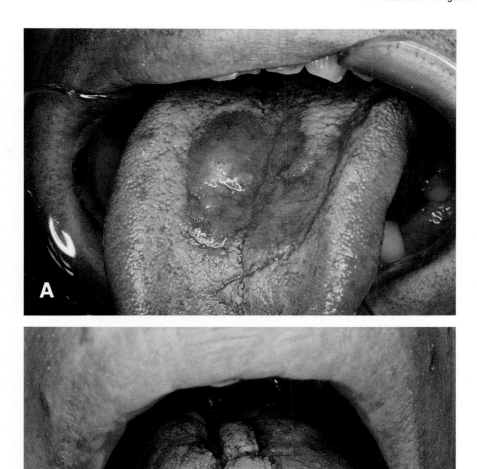

Figure 6.9 (A) Kaposi's sarcoma involving the tongue. (B) Kaposi's sarcoma occurring as "non-vascular"-appearing nodules.

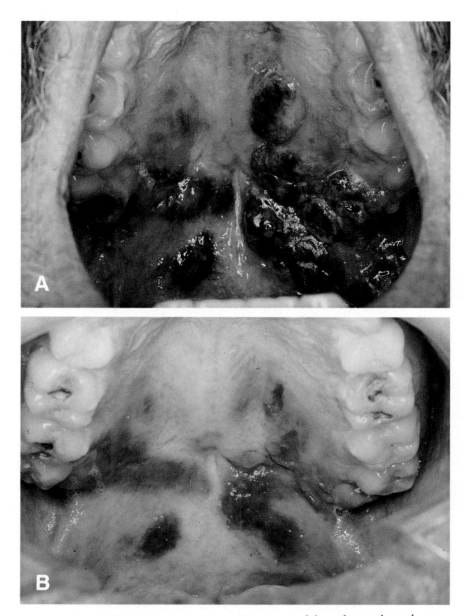

Figure 6.10 (A) Painful extensive Kaposi's sarcoma of the palate and oropharynx. (B) Remission of signs and symptoms following radiation therapy (1500 cGy in 10 days).

The most effective treatment for oral KS is low dose radiation, usually approximating 1500 cGy in 10 fractions (Figure 6.10). While this is not curative, it almost always reverses signs and symptoms. Excision (most effectively with laser) and chemotherapy with vinblastine have been useful in limited situations (Figures 6.11 and 6.12).

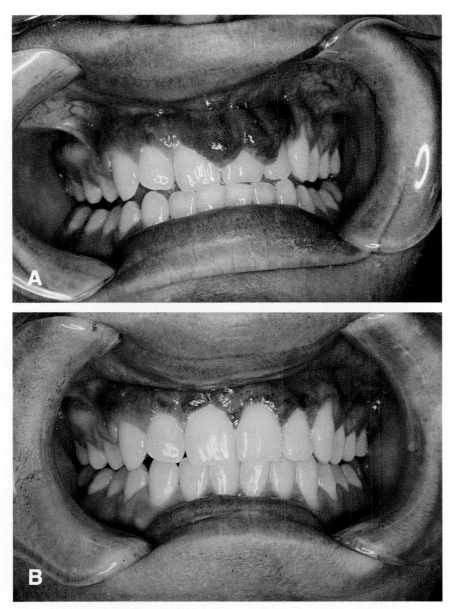

Figure 6.11 (A) Painful and esthetically undesirable Kaposi's sarcoma of the gingiva. (B) Three weeks following removal by CO_2 laser.

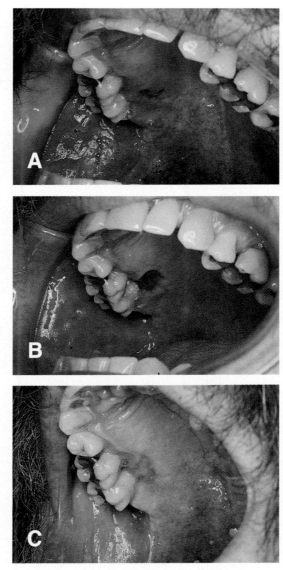

Figure 6.12 (A) Painful biopsy-proved Kaposi's sarcoma of the palate. (B) Appearance two weeks after an intralesional injection of vinblastine (0.6 mg). (C) Three months after injection, the lesion remains in remission.

LYMPHOMAS

The fastest growing number of malignancies in HIV-infected persons are lymphomas, with non-Hodgkin's lymphoma (NHL) being the most common form. Cofactors, in addition to immunosuppression, are unknown, although Epstein-Barr virus is suspect. Most cases appear to be extranodal. In some patients, NHL can occur first or only in the mouth (Figures 6.13 and 6.14). Therefore, when oral NHL tumors are found in patients, HIV infection and immunosuppression must be considered as possible causative factors. NHL is the most common malignancy seen in intravenous drug abusers with AIDS.

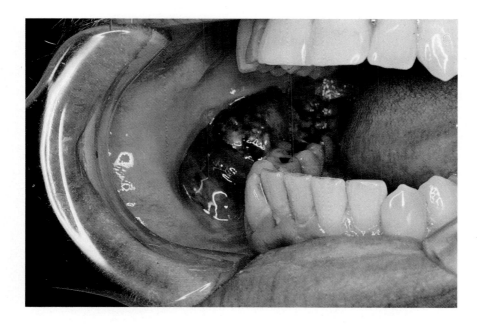

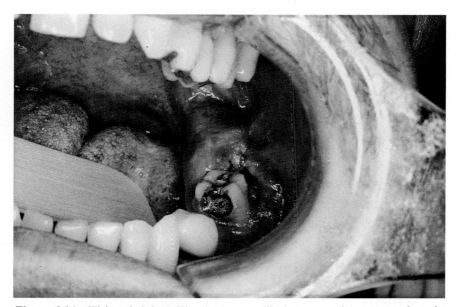

Figure 6.14   This painful swelling in the mandibular retromolar area was thought to be due to a dental abscess in this 30 year old homosexual nurse. When there was no response to antibiotics, a biopsy was obtained which revealed non-Hodgkin's lymphoma. The patient expired from disseminated disease four months later. He was HIV positive.

CARCINOMA

Oral squamous carcinomas occur primarily in individuals beyond their fourth decade of life. In HIV-infected young homosexual men, we have found squamous carcinomas more frequently than would be expected for this age group. The cause is uncertain, since immunosuppression could not be confirmed in all patients at the time of diagnosis. Tongue was by far the most common site, and a history of smoking, alcohol use, hepatitis B, and candidiasis was almost universal (Figures 6.15 to 6.17).

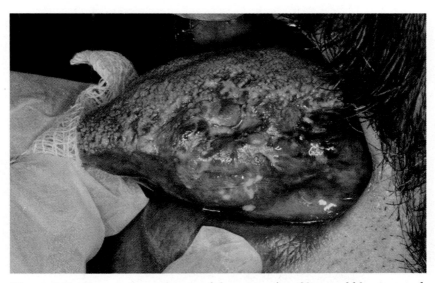

Figure 6.15   Squamous carcinoma of the tongue in a 30 year old homosexual man. He also was a moderately heavy smoker and drinker. Two years later he was shown to be HIV-infected.

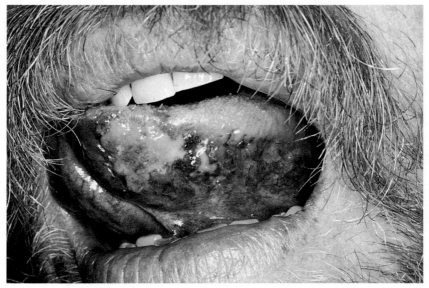

Figure 6.16   A 32 year old bisexual male with a two year history of erosive erythroplasia of the tongue. The anterior portion of the lesion revealed squamous carcinoma. The patient also had a history of venereal disease, hepatitis, and marijuana abuse.

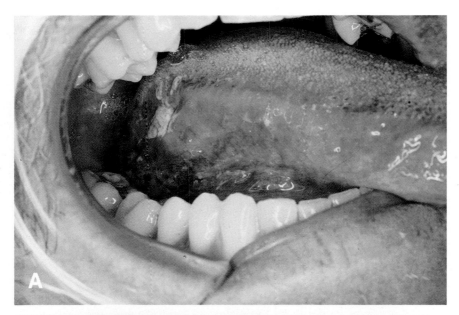

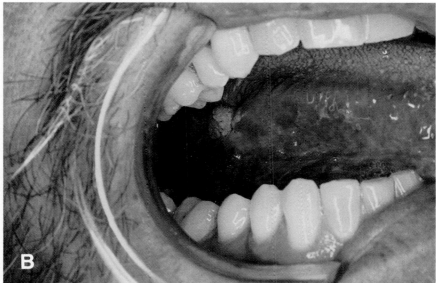

Figure 6.17   (A) A 26 year old homosexual man sought consultation because of a mild irritation of the right posterior tongue. A moderately firm erythroplastic lesion was noted inferior to an area of leukoplakia. His history was positive for venereal disease, hepatitis, and candidiasis. (B) The erythematous portion of the lesion retained stain after an application of 1 percent toluidine blue dye, and resisted decolorization with 1 percent acetic acid. A biopsy from the erythroplasia revealed squamous carcinoma.

REFERENCES

Kaposi's Sarcoma

Ficarra G, Benson AM, Silverman S Jr, et al. Kaposi's sarcoma of the oral cavity: a study of 134 patients with a review of the pathogenesis, epidemiology, clinical aspects, and treatment. Oral Surg Oral Med Oral Pathol 1988; 66:543–550.

Garrett TJ, Lange M, Ashford A, Thomas L. Kaposi's sarcoma in heterosexual intravenous drug users. Cancer 1985; 55:1146–1148.

Green TL, Beckstead JH, Lozada-Nur F, et al. Histopathology spectrum of oral Kaposi's sarcoma. Oral Surg Oral Med Oral Pathol 1984; 58:306–314.

Lumerman H, Freedman PD, Kerpel SM, Phelan JA. Oral Kaposi's sarcoma: a clinicopathologic study of 23 homosexual and bisexual men from the New York metropolitan area. Oral Surg Oral Med Oral Pathol 1988; 65:711–716.

Newland JR, Lynch DP, Ordonez NG. Intraoral Kaposi's sarcoma: a correlated light microscopic, ultrastructural, and immunohistochemical study. Oral Surg Oral Med Oral Pathol 1988; 66:48–58.

Lymphomas

Ahmed T, Wormser GP, Stahl RE, et al. Malignant lymphomas in a population at risk for acquired immune deficiency syndrome. Cancer 1987; 60:719–723.

Green TL, Eversole LR. Oral lymphomas in HIV-infected patients: associated with Epstein-Barr virus DNA. Oral Surg Oral Med Oral Pathol 1989; 67:437–442.

Ioachim HL, Cooper MC, Hellman GC. Lymphomas in men at high risk of acquired immune deficiency syndrome (AIDS). A study of 21 cases. Cancer 1985; 56:2831–2842.

Kaugers GE, Burns JC. Non-Hodgkin's lymphoma of the oral cavity associated with AIDS. Oral Surg Oral Med Oral Pathol 1989; 67:433–436.

Lowenthal DA, Straus DJ, Campbell SW, et al. AIDS-related lymphoid neoplasia. Cancer 1988; 61:2325–2337.

Carcinomas/HIV-Associated Malignancies

Eskinazi DP. Oncogenic potential of sexually transmitted viruses with special reference to oral cancer. Oral Surg Oral Med Oral Pathol 1987; 64:35–40.

Silverman S Jr, Migliorati CA, Lozada-Nur F, et al. Oral findings in people with or at high risk for AIDS: a study of 375 homosexual males. JADA 1986; 112:187–192.

7

OTHER HIV-ASSOCIATED MANIFESTATIONS

H IV infection-associated pathology has brought about a multitude of new, complex, and diverse signs and symptoms that have complicated diagnoses and posed significant management problems. Some of the conditions are new and as yet not clearly classified, and many other lesions are known "seen before" entities that occur more frequently and/or in more severe forms. Obviously, successful treatment depends upon a correct diagnosis, knowledge of therapeutic approaches, and host factors, most prominent being the stage of HIV infection (status of immune competence).

RECURRENT APHTHOUS STOMATITIS

All data at present indicate that recurrent aphthous stomatitis (RAS) is a manifestation of an autoimmune abnormality. Ordinarily, these ulcerations occur in about 20 to 40 percent of the general population, depending upon the target study group. In HIV-infected individuals, there appears to be an increased frequency in persons having RAS attacks for the first time. In those with previous RAS histories, attacks are more frequent or severe (Figure 7.1). Severity is often reflected as either multiple-lesion occurrences or major aphthae. Major aphthae infer lesions that exceed 6 mm in diameter, persist for longer periods of time, and are usually quite painful (Figure 7.2).

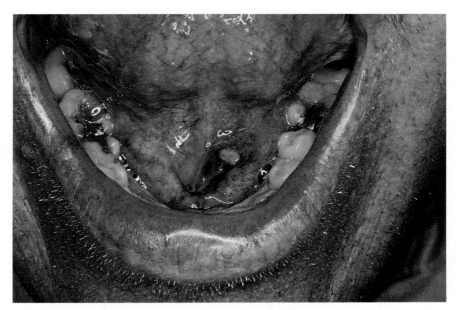

Figure 7.1 A painful minor aphthous ulcer in an HIV-infected patient who had no prior history of aphthae.

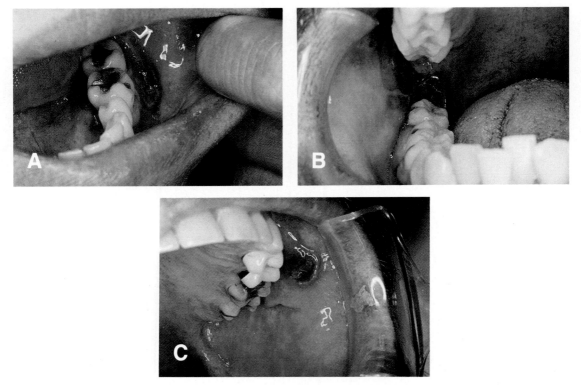

Figure 7.2 Major aphthae in otherwise asymptomatic HIV-positive patients. These large aphthae persist for months, are very painful and usually require anti-inflammatory corticosteroid treatment for effective control. (A) Buccal-gingival reflex. (B) Mandibular retromolar gingiva. (C) Buccal mucosa.

The diagnosis of RAS can often be established on the basis of history and appearance. However, because of the size, induration, and duration of major aphthae, carcinoma and granulomatous diseases related to microbial infections may be considered in the differential diagnosis. Therefore, biopsy sometimes is indicated.

Treatment is often mandatory because of pain and difficulty in eating (Figure 7.3). Alterations in food intake can lead to marked weight loss, which adds to an already compromised immune status and "resistance." RAS treatment is directed against the lymphocytes associated with the lesions. By far the most effective approach entails the use of corticosteroids. Systemic approaches involve the use of prednisone. Daily dosages usually vary between 40 to 60 mg. The duration of therapy is determined by cessation of symptoms or signs. Adequate responses usually occur in less than 2 weeks, which eliminates the need for tapering. In our studies short-term administration of prednisone has not complicated or affected the immune suppression status.

Topical corticosteroid usage involves application of ointments such as 0.05 percent fluocinonide or 0.05 percent clobetasol mixed with equal parts of orabase, or daily mouth rinses (1 minute swish and empty) with an elixir of dexamethasone.

HYPERSENSITIVITY, LICHENOID REACTIONS

As indicated previously, at least 40 percent of HIV-infected individuals have central nervous system involvement, which may increase to 75 percent by the terminal phase of infection. There is an indication of pituitary involvement and decreased daily production of endogenous (adrenal cortex) cortisone. This phenomenon, in addition to immune system suppression, may add to and aggravate the increase of acquired allergies experienced by those that are HIV infected. Many of these hypersensitivities are autoimmune, while others develop in response to medications and food (Figures 7.4 to 7.7).

Diagnosis is primarily based on history and clinical findings, but cultures or smears and biopsy are often helpful to rule out other conditions. Management involves the following: identification of allergens and avoidance; prevention by use of antihistamines; and definitive treatment by the use of systemic or topical corticosteroids. Anaphylaxis is extremely rare.

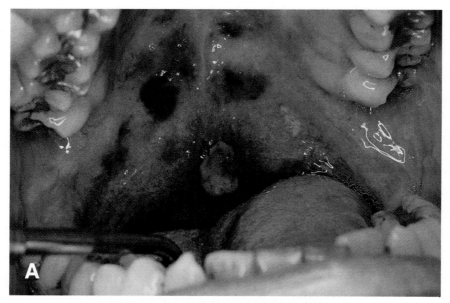

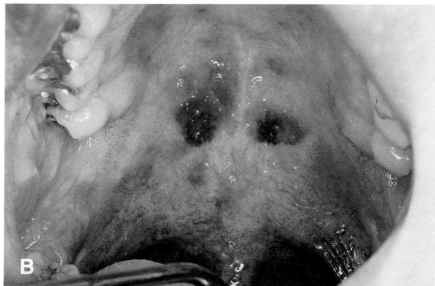

Figure 7.3   (A) This AIDS patient had Kaposi's sarcoma of the palate along with a major aphthous ulcer of soft palate, persisting for 2 weeks and "getting worse." Because of the pain, he was not eating and already had lost 12 pounds, which was further compromising his prognosis. He was stable prior to the ulcer. After three days of 60 mg prednisone daily, the symptoms were minimal and the patient was again eating. (B) After one week of treatment, the lesion had completely healed.

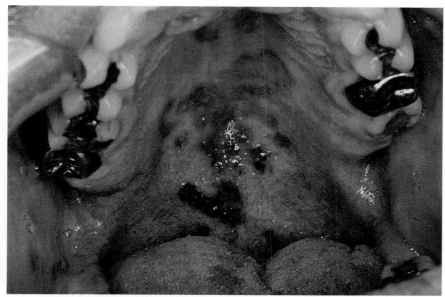

Figure 7.4   This HIV-positive homosexual male complained of progressive palatal pain of 2 weeks duration. The differential diagnosis included trauma, allergy (erythema multiforme), and infection (fungal, viral, or bacterial). Cultures were negative for any specific microbial pathogen. The patient was treated with prednisone on a presumptive working diagnosis of erythema multiforme. The lesions cleared in 3 days.

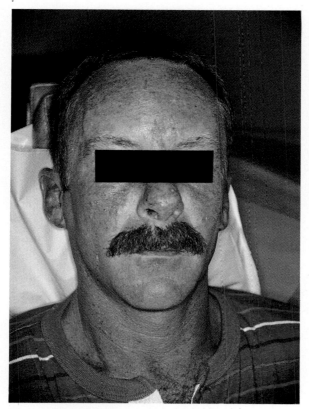

Figure 7.5   This HIV-infected patient was asymptomatic except for oral candidiasis. Ketoconazole therapy (200 mg daily) cleared the oral signs and symptoms, but led to a severe facial skin rash. This cleared on drug withdrawal, and recurred when the drug was used again subsequently, confirming a hypersensitivity to ketoconazole.

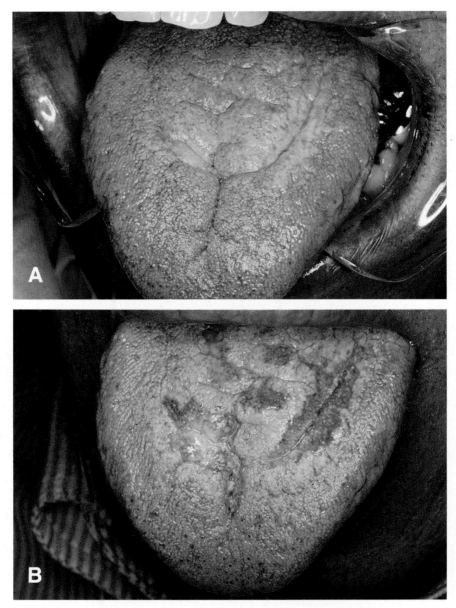

Figure 7.6   (A) This 36 year old homosexual man who had been HIV infected for 2 years developed oral discomfort. The tongue lesion was biopsied and found to be clinically and histologically consistent with lichen planus. Culture of the mouth and special staining of the biopsy specimen revealed no evidence of candida. (B) The lesion has persisted for more than one year and periodically becomes erythematous (atrophic form of lichen planus).

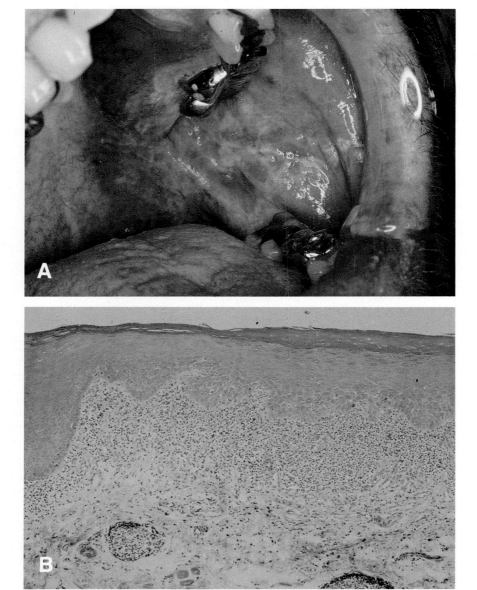

Figure 7.7 (A) This AIDS patient with Kaposi's sarcoma of the palate developed asymptomatic reticular keratoses of the buccal mucosa and palate. There was no evident causative factor. (B) A biopsy revealed a lichenoid-type reaction.

THROMBOCYTOPENIA

Paradoxically, one antibody that many HIV-infected persons produce is a protein directed against their own blood platelets. When this event occurs, which can be early in HIV infection, platelet counts may drop from normal values above 200,000 to 300,000 per mm³ of blood to around 100,000 or less. At this level, there may be spontaneous or easily-induced bruising (ecchymosis), or some clotting problems after injury (Figure 7.8). In some cases, counts will drop well below 50,000, which incurs greater problems including spontaneous bleeding from the mouth, hematomas, and bleeding control following dental and oral procedures.

Treatment measures may require corticosteroids, transfusions, and splenectomy.

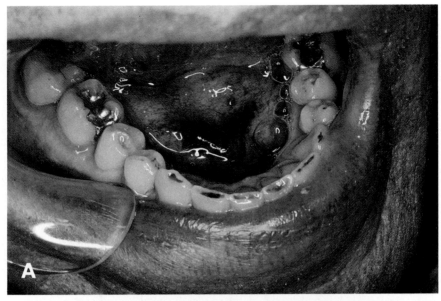

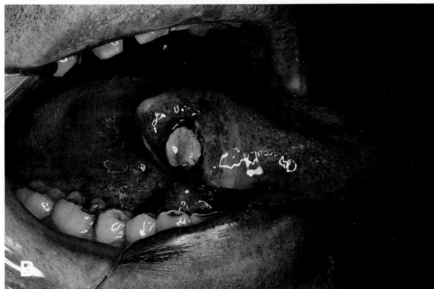

Figure 7.8   (A) This HIV-positive drug abuser had generalized toxoplasmosis with central nervous system involvement. His platelet count was less than 50,000 per mm³. Note the purpuric lesion in the floor of his mouth (thrombocytopenic purpura). (B) During a seizure he bit his tongue, inducing a necrotic ulcer and hematoma.

SIALADENITIS, XEROSTOMIA

Frequently, HIV-infected patients complain of an oral dryness, which often can be documented by a decreased salivary flow rate. The cause is unknown, but may be due to an autoimmune reaction or cytomegalovirus (CMV) infection and subsequent salivary gland inflammation. CMV presence in HIV-infected individuals is common, and CMV salivary gland predilection is known.

Enlargement of the major salivary glands may occur without apparent reason (Figure 7.9). However, it is not usually associated with xerostomia, but it does raise concern for establishing a cause and diagnosis, and consideration of treatment for discomfort or appearance. The differential diagnoses of salivary gland enlargement must include infection, tumor, and inflammation. Approaches most commonly include a trial with antibiotics to rule out infection, and a fine needle aspiration biopsy to rule out neoplasia (especially lymphoma). The most frequent finding is that of idiopathic benign hyperplasia.

Management in benign conditions is usually directed towards keeping the mouth comfortably moist. This approach entails frequent mouth rinses, sugarless candy or gum, salivary substitutes, and salivary gland stimulants (pilocarpine or bethanechol). Follow-up is important because of the possibility of transformations to malignancy or acute, painful flares. Since a viral etiology has not been shown, it is expected that salivary gland enlargement has not responded to antiviral drugs. Antibiotics and anti-inflammatory medicines have been equally ineffective.

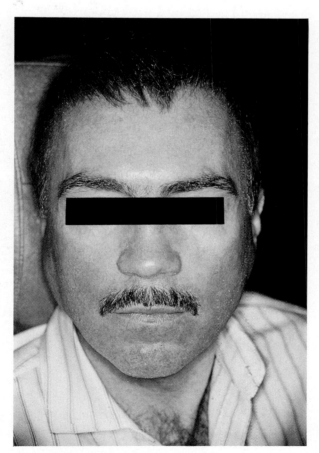

Figure 7.9 This HIV-infected patient had mildly symptomatic, chronic, bilateral parotid gland swelling for more than two years. Cultures were negative for any infectious microbial organism and a fine needle aspiration biopsy was negative for lymphoma. Causative factors and long-term prognosis are unknown. Treatment is symptomatic. This might represent an auto-immune inflammatory salivary gland response.

UNCLASSIFIED ORAL LESIONS

It is quite common that HIV-infected patients will seek consultation regarding signs and symptoms that do not lend themselves to an obvious diagnosis or indication of an etiologic agent (Figures 7.10 to 7.11). Many times a series of laboratory tests, and even biopsy, do not shed light on the classification, with the only resultant value being that of ruling out known neoplastic and infectious diseases. Treatment therefore becomes one of palliation, empirical trials, and follow up.

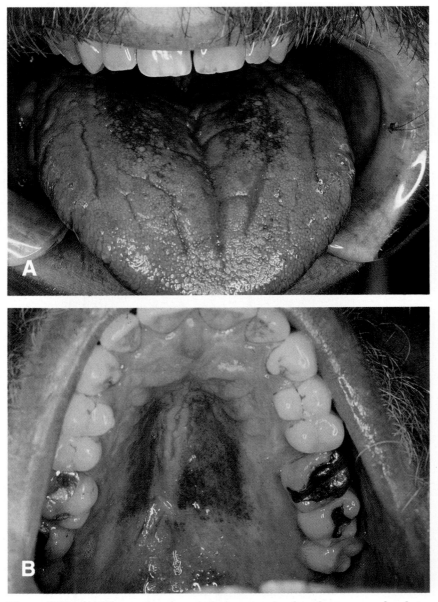

Figure 7.10   (A) These telangiectatic lesions on the dorsal tongue and palate (B) were asymptomatic and chronic; they have been present consistently for more than one year without change in this AIDS patient. A biopsy showed a nonspecific mucositis and all other tests were non-contributory. Also, there was no correlation between medical status or habits. The significance of these not-too-infrequent mucosal changes is unknown.

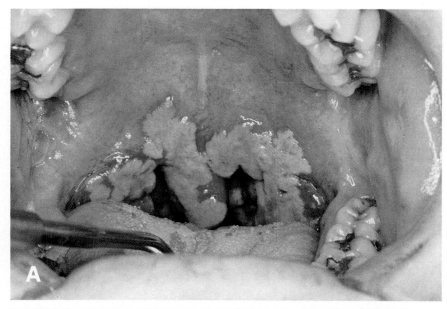

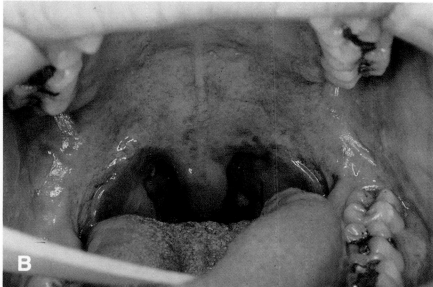

Figure 7.11   (A) This oropharyngeal pseudomembranous lesion was present without change in this 26 year old HIV-positive patient for four months. Cultures were negative for virus, candida, or predominant bacterial pathogens. A biopsy revealed a non-specific mucositis. No treatment was instituted because the lesion did not bother the patient. (B) All signs spontaneously disappeared during the fifth month.

REFERENCES

Lozada-Nur F, Gorsky M, Silverman S Jr. Oral erythema multiforme: clinical observations and treatment in fifty-five patients. Oral Surg Oral Med Oral Pathol 1989; 67:36–40.

Morris L, Distenfeld A, Amorosi E, Karpatkin S. Autoimmune thrombocytopenia purpura in homosexual men. Ann Intern Med 1982; 96:714–717.

Pindborg JJ. Classification of oral lesions associated with HIV infections. Oral Surg Oral Med Oral Pathol 1989; 67:292–295.

Silverman S Jr, Lozada-Nur F, Migliorati C. Clinical efficacy of prednisone in the treatment of patients with oral inflammatory ulcerative diseases: a study of fifty-five patients. Oral Surg Oral Med Oral Pathol 1985; 59:360–363.

Ulirsch RC, Jaffe ES. Sjögren's syndrome-like illness associated with the acquired immunodeficiency syndrome-related complex. Hum Pathol 1987; 18:1063–1068.

8

CASE PRESENTATIONS

T he purpose of this chapter is to illustrate both the variety of signs and symptoms found within individual HIV-infected patients and the progression of disease. Dental professionals frequently participate in the diagnosis and share treatment responsibilities that often involve counseling and appropriate referrals. An understanding of oral AIDS, participation in management, and some compassion for the afflicted can contribute to improving the existing quality of life.

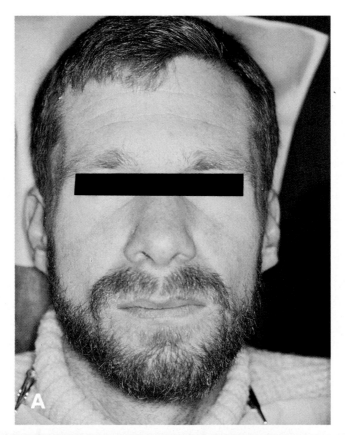

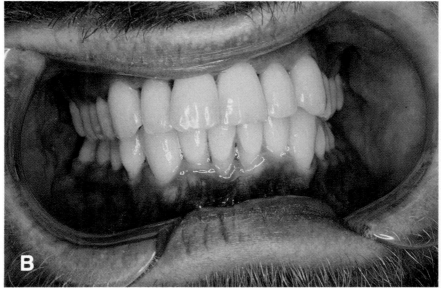

Figure 8.1 (A) This apparently healthy 27 year old man reported to the clinic with a chief complaint of mildly sore gums. Medical history included hepatitis B and venereal infections, and sporadic use of cocaine, marijuana, amyl nitrate, and alcohol. He had experienced no previous weight loss, malaise, or night sweats. (B) Findings included gingival recession and alveolar bone loss involving teeth #24 and #25 in particular, and blunted-ulcerated interdental papilla. Hygiene was good.

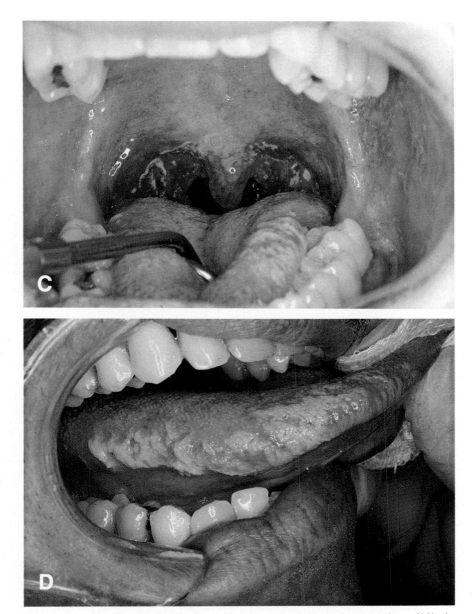

Figure 8.1 *Continued.* Further examination revealed oropharyngeal candidiasis, (C) and hairy leukoplakia, (D). Laboratory tests showed positive HIV serology and skin anergy to four antigens (candida, PPD, mumps, trichophyton).

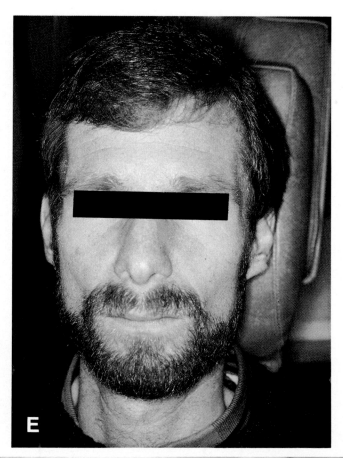

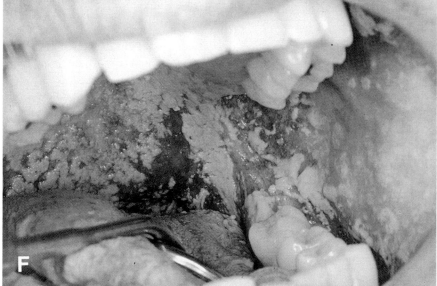

Figure 8.1 *Continued.* (E) Four months later he had lost 30 pounds, developed *Pneumocystis carinii* pneumonia with severe dyspnea, and experienced progressive weakness and malaise. One month later his oral candidiasis had become florid (F) and refractive to treatment, his T4 lymphocytes fell below 50 per mm^3, and he expired the following month.

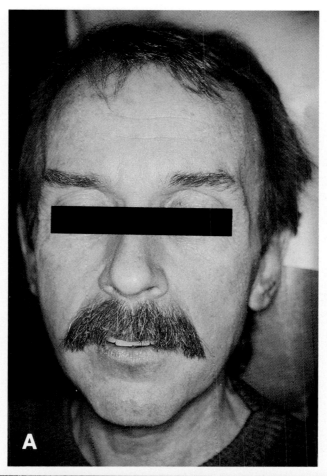

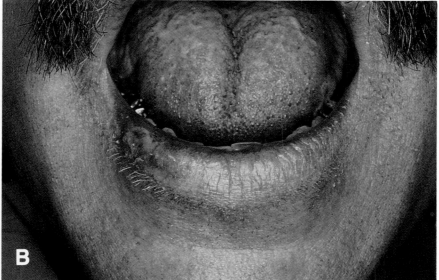

Figure 8.2   (A) This 34 year old AIDS patient complained of dental pain. He has had Kaposi's sarcoma for 1 year, with one bout of *Pneumocystis carinii* pneumonia and some recurrent diarrhea. Examination confirmed herpes labialis (B).

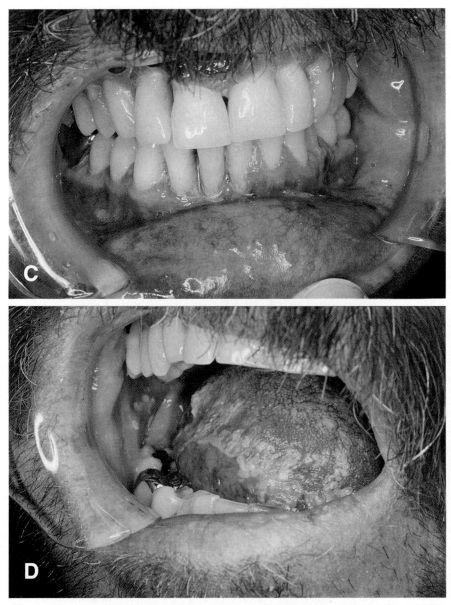

Figure 8.2 *Continued.*   Examination also confirmed advanced dental disease (C), hairy leukoplakia (D) and Kaposi's sarcoma.

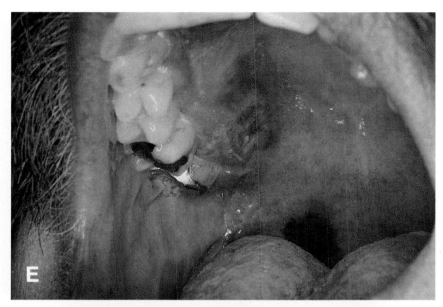

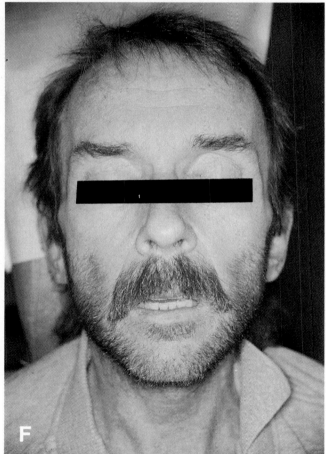

Figure 8.2 *Continued.* (E) He returned 2 weeks later for selected extractions, but rapid weight loss, extreme malaise, and weakness precluded any dental work (F). He expired 2 weeks later.

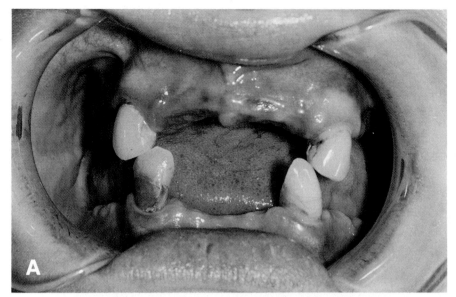

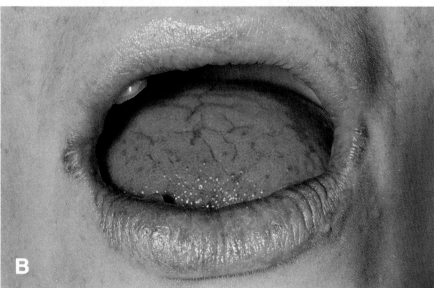

Figure 8.3   This 32 year old heterosexual female drug addict has been asymptomatic and known to be HIV positive for 2 years. She currently is on methadone control and seeking prosthodontic care (A). She had recently developed symptomatic oral candidiasis. Note the angular cheilitis (B).

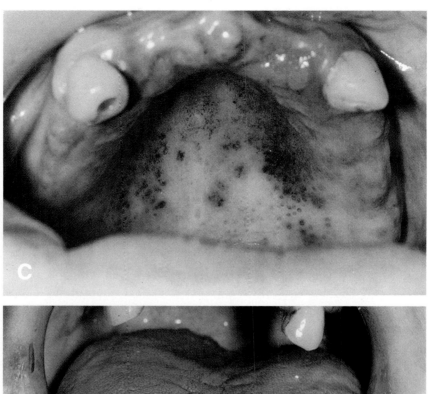

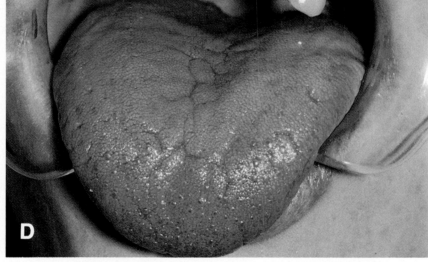

Figure 8.3 *Continued.*   Note also the telangiectatic-appearing palatal candidiasis (C). Her tongue was also mildly depapillated and sensitive (D). A fungal culture showed heavy growth of *Candida albicans*, which has presently responded to ketoconazole. Her T4 lymphocytes are below 400 per mm³. Of utmost importance, she is in need of counseling. She has an HIV-negative live-in partner who does not use barrier techniques, and she now wants a baby. Obviously, both her partner and baby are at risk of becoming HIV positive, and her prognosis for survival is poor.

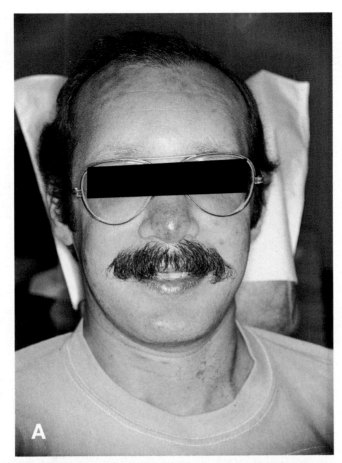

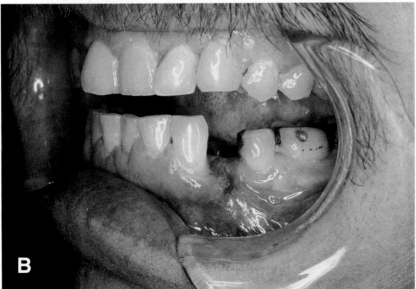

Figure 8.4 This 32 year old street artist presented to the clinic because of a "tooth ache" in his edentulous lower left first bicuspid area (A). Otherwise he claimed to be in good health and jogged daily. The vascular-appearing lesions and nodules on the skin of his head and neck were characteristic of Kaposi's sarcoma. Intraoral examination revealed an early Kaposi's involving the area of his chief complaint, (B). He was counseled regarding his condition, which was confirmed by serology and biopsy. He was referred to the adult immunodeficiency clinic for further evaluation.

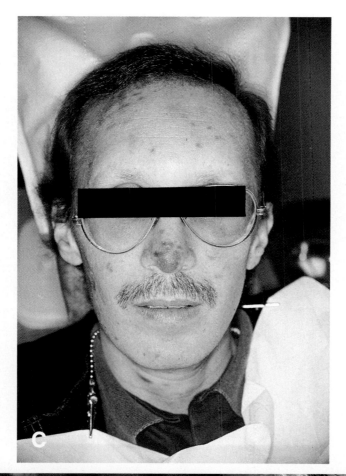

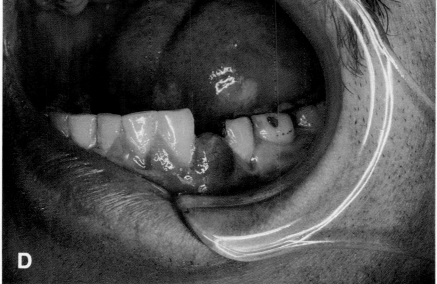

Figure 8.4 *Continued.* Three months later immunosuppression progressed rapidly, leaving him markedly cachectic and weak, (C). His intraoral Kaposi's progressed and became more bothersome (D). He expired 2 months later.

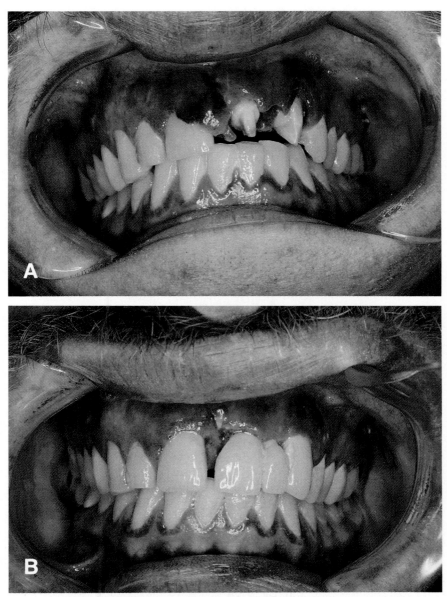

Figure 8.5   This AIDS patient had just lost his anterior bridge. Note the Kaposi's sarcoma of the maxilla, and HIV-associated gingivitis of the mandibular marginal gingiva, (A). The Kaposi's was excised and the bridge recemented, (B). The patient survived for an additional 6 months.

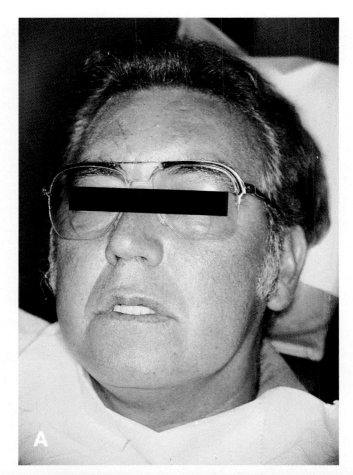

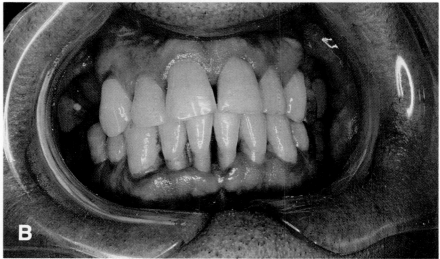

Figure 8.6   (A) This 42 year old bisexual man sought consultation because of a chronically sore mouth for 4 months. He was recently married and had a young daughter, but admitted to previous homosexual activities. (B) He had periodontosis in spite of a good record of home and office care.

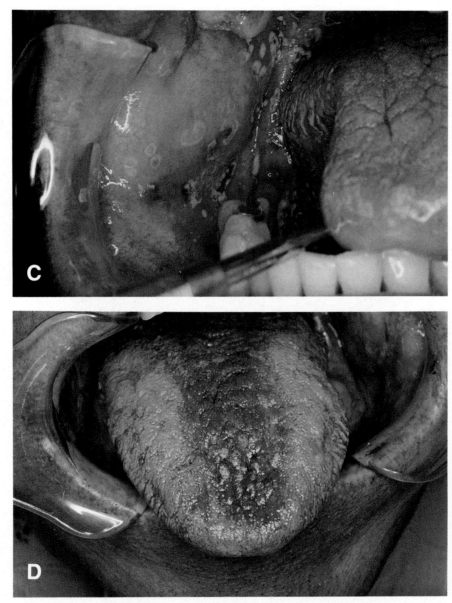

Figure 8.6 *Continued.*   (C and D) Clinical and laboratory examinations confirmed buccal (pseudomembranous and hypertrophic) and tongue (erythematous, atrophic) lesions of candidiasis. When treated with antifungal medications, both signs and symptoms disappeared.

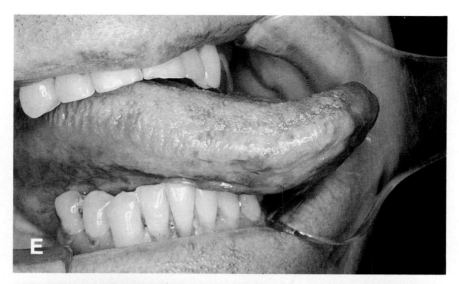

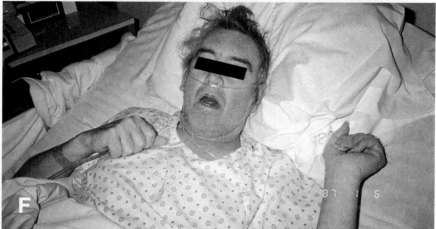

Figure 8.6 *Continued.* Hairy leukoplakia was confirmed by biopsy and persisted during antifungal treatment. (E), He was surprised when his serology was HIV positive. During the following year, his response to antifungal treatment became increasingly refractory. He also developed severe anal candidiasis and intraepithelial carcinoma of the glans penis. He began losing weight rapidly, had bouts of protozoal diarrhea, and developed *Pneumocystis carinii* pneumonia with severe malaise and depression. He and his family asked not to have life support systems, and he died during his second week of hospitalization, (F).

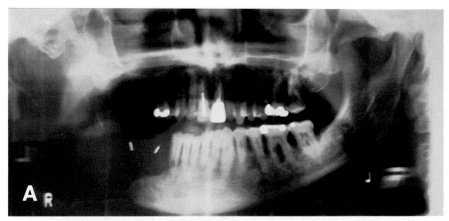

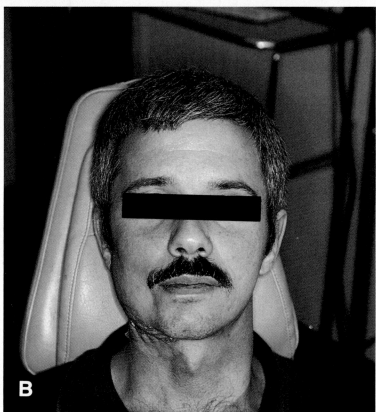

Figure 8.7   A 27 year old homosexual man developed a squamous carcinoma of the right lateral tongue in 1977. He had a history of hepatitis B, syphilis and gonorrhea, and herpes. He did not use tobacco, alcohol, or "recreational" drugs. Although his tumor responded to radiation therapy, he developed osteonecrosis of his right mandible that did not respond to treatment. Two years later he had a resection (A). Note also the periodontal disease. His chronic candidiasis was thought to be due to constant use of antibiotics. (B) During this period the patient felt well, so 1 year after the resection, he had a muscle graft to improve appearance.

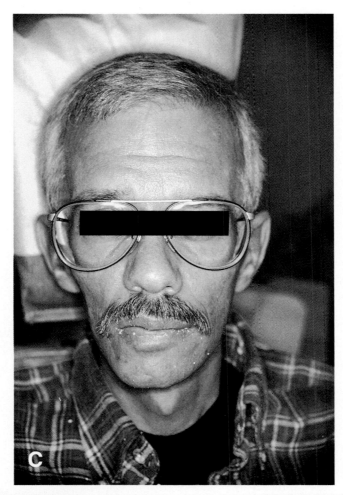

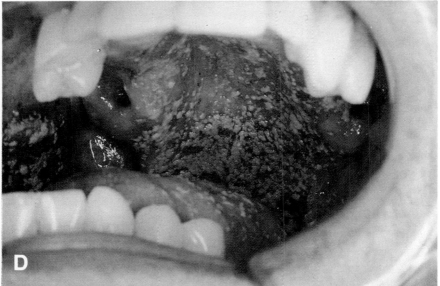

Figure 8.7 *Continued.* Four years later, he suddenly developed progressive weight loss, treatment-resistant oral candidiasis, and extreme mobility of teeth and pain, (C and D). HIV infection was confirmed. The aging process was marked. In a short period of time *Pneumocystis carinii* pneumonia was diagnosed and the patient died. There were no specimens that enabled review of HIV status prior to the progressive wasting syndrome features. Therefore, immunosuppression at the time of his early-onset carcinoma can only be speculated.

Index

15